Communicating Health

An action guide to health education and health promotion

Second edition

John Hubley

...municating Health: An Action Guide to Health
Education and Health Promotion

2nd
Oxford: Macmillan, 2004   1405028831

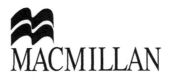

MACMILLAN

Macmillan Education
Between Towns Road, Oxford ox4 3pp
A division of Macmillan Publishers Limited
Companies and representatives throughout the world

www.macmillan-africa.com
www.macmillan-caribbean.com

ISBN 978-1-4050-2883-7

Text © John Hubley 2004
Design and illustration © Macmillan Publishers Limited 2004

First edition 1993
Second edition 2004

Designed by Jim Weaver Design
Typeset by EXPO Holdings, Malaysia
Cover design by Wheeler and Porter
Cover photographs clockwise: school child in China; scene
from a video on patient education in Namibia with an actor
playing the role of patient in an imaginary setting (Photo also
used on back cover); a training workshop on participatory
learning materials in Ghana and pre-testing of a flip-chart in
Nigeria. Photographs by the author with grateful thanks to
those appearing in the photographs.

Printed and bound in Malaysia

2008 2007
10 9 8 7 6 5 4 3 2

Contents

Introduction

The purpose of this revised and updated book remains the same as in the first edition. It is aimed at those of you who find yourselves in a position where you are having to plan programmes to improve the health of your communities. I hope to present you with a 'state of the art' view of the best of what is currently practised in developing countries as well as approaches from industrialised countries. While the book is based on theory and proven research, I have kept it at a simple level and those of you who wish to explore issues further can use the further reading and links provided at the end of the book and web site listed below.

Ten years have passed since the publication of the first edition of *Communicating Health*. Preparing a new edition is a time of reflection and rethinking of priorities. In one respect the situation has not changed since the first edition. Health promotion, health education and the prevention of disease continue to pose important challenges. Some interesting new developments have taken place and I have included these in this new edition. Alongside these new developments, there is a need to restate the principles of communication planning that I set out in the first edition. A renewed interest by donors and international agencies in supporting health promotion is starting to bear fruit and I have been able to expand the number of examples of successful programmes that have applied those principles.

One of the most important developments in recent years has been that of the concept of evidence-based practice. Following the first edition, I began to receive questions from colleagues asking for evidence for the effectiveness of health education. That led to the setting up of the Leeds Health Education Database of evaluated interventions in developing countries. This proved an exciting and worthwhile experience because it brought together for the first time the proof that health education in developing countries has progressed to a mature discipline. Good evidence now exists for the contribution it can play to improvement in health in developing countries. The database is an ongoing project and is updated regularly and is posted on my personal web site listed below. A series of case studies drawn from the database is an important new feature of this edition.

The overall structure of the book is shown on page ix. Chapter 1 introduces health education and health promotion and Chapters 2–4 act as core chapters. Further details of particular methods are given in Chapters 5–10 and the final chapter provides guidelines on planning, evaluation and implementation. You should look upon the content of this book as guidelines rather than a set of rules. What may work in one community may not work in another. But if you apply these methods in a systematic way, involve the communities you are working with, evaluate and learn from mistakes, you should be able to improve the effectiveness of your activities.

The amount of information that can be provided in a book of this short length is inevitably limited. For those wishing to read further, I have prepared an appendix with a list of some key books supplied by TALC (Teaching aids At Low Cost). I have given details of a range of newsletters and journals, many of which are free to persons from developing countries. I have also provided addresses of resource agencies that might be able to help you in your work.

One of the most significant developments since the first edition has been the rise of the Internet, which opens up a vast resource of knowledge and experience. I have provided details of some of the more important Internet web sites. However a unique feature of this book is the establishment of a web site dedicated exclusively to serving the needs of the reader. I plan to use this web site to provide supporting information, regularly updated links to other sites and details of the case studies that feature in this new edition. I am aware that some of you are trainers and use this book as a resource for your students. The web site provides a set of teaching resources including exercises and PowerPoint presentations that are linked to specific chapters of the book. Finally, the web site is a mechanism for including feedback from readers. I would be happy to hear from you about the work you are doing and receive comments on this book. Good luck in your work!

Dr John Hubley
www.hubley.co.uk
www.communicatinghealth.com

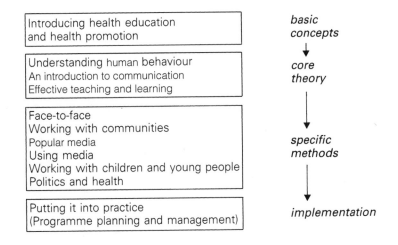

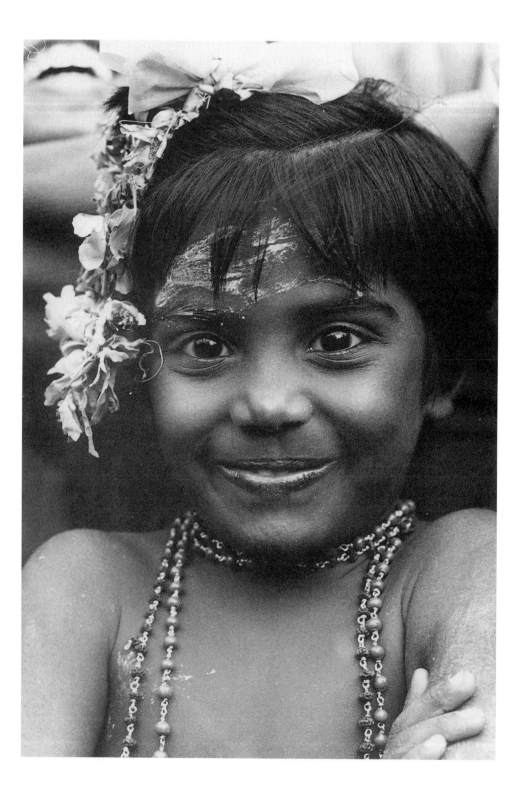

Acknowlegements

I would like to acknowledge the ideas and support received from a number of persons: the students on the various health education courses I have taught and learned so much from at Leeds and at the various workshops I have facilitated in other countries; my colleagues at Leeds who have provided so much stimulation and so many ideas, especially June Copeman, John Mee, Maggie Holt, Professor Keith Tones and Dr Rachael Dixey.

I would also like to acknowledge the inspiration and stimulation provided by Professor David Morley and Dr Felicity Savage King whose encouragement was so important in preparing the original edition.

Thanks also to Vikasbhai, Harry Dickinson, Ken Cripwell and Dr Peter Cox. In their different ways all four had significant influence on my thinking about health and development and their deaths were a great loss.

I would like to thank the various health educators with whom I have had the privilege of working or exchanging ideas, including: Professor Joshua Adeniyi, Dr Khalifa Bility, Marieke Boot, Dr Bill Brieger, Ann Burgess, Susan Durston, Ane Haaland, Dr Anita Hardon, Dr Saroj Jha, Dr Glenn Laverack, George McBean, Dr Chandra Mouli, Martha Osei, Dr Kathy Parker, Jean Ritchie, Hazel Slavin, Dr Peter Sternberg, Dr Benchung Tiang and Kathy Wolfheim.

Special thanks go to Dr Pat Pridmore for her useful suggestions of topics for inclusion in the new edition.

While many of the ideas in this book were obtained while working as consultant in Africa, the Caribbean, Asia and the Pacific for WHO, UNICEF, the EU, DANIDA and DFID, the ideas in this book do not represent the views of any of these agencies. The responsibility for any mistakes or inaccuracies is entirely my own.

And finally, thanks to my wife Penny. Our mutual concerns over the issues of poverty and health in the developing world had brought us together. She was a constant companion in shaping my ideas and supporting me in my work. Together we took most of the photographs in this book. She supported and encouraged me through the lengthy process of preparing the first edition. Her untimely death from breast cancer was a great blow. I miss her greatly.

Illustrations and photographs

Grateful acknowledgement is made to: WHO South East Asia Region for permission to use illustrations from their manual *Achieving Success in Water and Sanitation*; Ministry of Health, Republic of Fiji for use of illustrations from their *Handbook on Health*; WHO CDD programme for illustration from the *Communication Manager's Guide*; WHO for the illustration on patient education and immunisation; Healthlink (formerly ARHTAG) for permission to use the illustration by Paul Cook on programme planning; UNICEF in Nepal for use of illustrations from their visual literacy studies and handbook of illustrations and fortune-teller's card; UNICEF EAPRO Regional Headquarters in Bankok for permission to use cartoons; *Action* comic; Pitnera Mthembu, Ministry of Health, Swaziland; Ministry of Health Sri Lanka, for leaflet; Dr Patrick Johnson of the Population Communication Institute, Johns Hopkins University for photograph of Tatiana and Johnny; Professor David Morley for several illustrations from *My Name is Today* and *Paediatric Priorities*; Dr Hermione Lovell for the illustration on the research process; Child-to-Child for the use of the illustration from *Toys for Fun*; John Pinfold and the Leeds University Thailand Hygiene Education Project for reproduction of a page of their storybook on hygiene; International Planned Parenthood Federation for several illustrations.

Every attempt has been made to trace and acknowledge the copyright owners of the illustrations in this book. If a mistake has been made please accept our apologies and we will make due amendments in a future printing.

The photographs on the cover and in the text are by the author with grateful thanks to the persons who appear in the photographs.

1 Introducing health education and health promotion

The aims of this chapter

A starting point for our look at health education and health promotion is the recognition that widespread disease represents a major cause of death, suffering and an obstacle to achieving health. This chapter will consider the following questions:

1   What are the main health problems and their contributory causes in developing countries?
2   What do we mean by health education and health promotion and why are they important for the prevention of disease and promotion of health?
3   What is the role of communication in supporting health promotion and health education?
4   What decisions do we have to make to plan and implement effective health education and health promotion programmes in our communities?

Health problems in developing countries

Children at risk

Children make up more than half the population in most developing countries. One in five children in the poorest parts of the world do not live beyond their fifth birthday. The main caus-es of death in this age group are malnutrition, diarrhoea and respiratory infections. The accumulated burden of low birthweight, malnutrition, diarrhoea, respiratory and other infections can result in death, stunting and failure to achieve mental and physical potential. This represents a tragic waste – *and most of the causes of death and disability can be prevented.*

Dangerous childbirth

In the poorest countries, the risk of dying from pregnancy and childbirth is 200 times higher than in developed countries. The reasons for maternal mortality are: high number of pregnancies, close spacing of births, lack of antenatal care, lack of access to family planning, unsafe abortion practices and teenage pregnancies. In response to these problems WHO launched a 'Safe Motherhood Programme'.

Water-related disease

The World Health Organization estimates that 80% of all sickness in the world is because of poor water and sanitation and reports that:

*   more than 3 million people – mostly children – die every year from water-related diseases;
*   1.1 billion people lack access to improved water sources;
*   2.4 billion people lack access to basic sanitation;

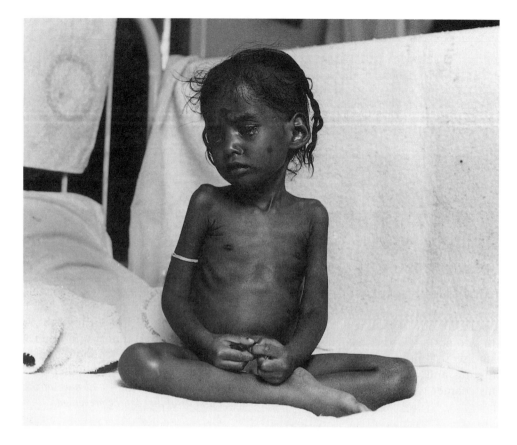

Priority health measures in Third World countries

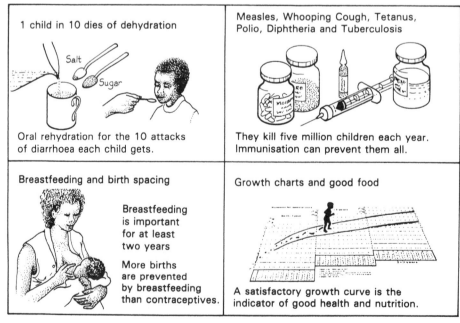

1 child in 10 dies of dehydration	Measles, Whooping Cough, Tetanus, Polio, Diphtheria and Tuberculosis
Oral rehydration for the 10 attacks of diarrhoea each child gets.	They kill five million children each year. Immunisation can prevent them all.
Breastfeeding and birth spacing	Growth charts and good food
Breastfeeding is important for at least two years. More births are prevented by breastfeeding than contraceptives.	A satisfactory growth curve is the indicator of good health and nutrition.

Fig. 1.1   Children are the priority group for health programmes in developing countries

- the daily task of collecting water represents a heavy burden on the women in developing countries affecting their own health as well as their ability to care for their families.

According to Bradley's environmental classification of water-related diseases, some of these infections are passed through drinking water as *water-borne diseases*. However, many are transmitted through contamination during collection and storage of the water as well as by contamination of hands, fingers and food. As water for practising hygiene is often the limiting factor, these are called *water-washed diseases*. In *water-based diseases* such as schistosomiasis, part of the parasite life cycle is in water. In the *water-related insect vector* diseases such as malaria, onchocerciasis and filariasis transmission of disease is by an insect that breeds in water.

Disability

One in ten persons in the world suffers from some form of disability such as blindness, physical impairment or injuries, resulting in loss of earning and discrimination. According to WHO there are an estimated 180 million people who are visually disabled, 40 million of whom are completely blind. Some 80% of global blindness can be avoided through prevention or simple treatment and unless there is urgent action the global burden of blindness will double by the year 2020. Some of the causes of blindness are complex and difficult to prevent, such as cataract and glaucoma, and the challenge is to increase access to treatment. Other causes such as onchocerciasis, trachoma, vitamin A deficiency, type 2 diabetes and injuries are clearly preventable.

Infectious and parasitic diseases

In developing countries the main disease burden comes from acute infectious diseases and malnutrition. In addition to the water-related diseases described above:

- Nearly three million people die each year

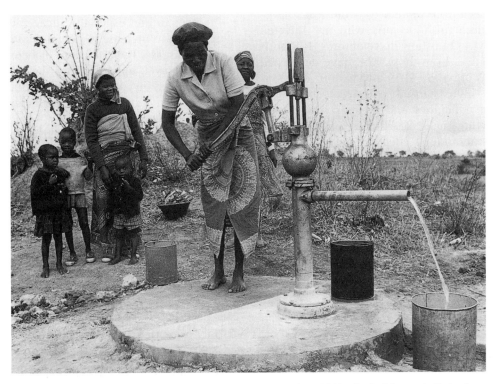

Fig. 1.2   The World Health Organization estimates that 80% of all sickness is linked to water and sanitation

from tuberculosis – most of whom are in the developing world.

- It is possible to immunise against many infectious diseases including measles, polio, pertussis, rubella, tuberculosis and tetanus. WHO estimates that more than 8000 children die each day because they are not immunised against vaccine-preventable diseases. Measles alone kills 1.4 million infants and tetanus kills 767,000 newborns a year.
- WHO estimated that in 2002 there would be over 10 million deaths in developing countries as a result of acute respiratory infections, diarrhoeal diseases, tuberculosis and malaria – all conditions for which safe, inexpensive and life-saving essential drugs exist but do not reach those who need them.

AIDS and other sexually-transmitted diseases

AIDS is an example of an infectious disease that is transmitted through sexual intercourse, blood products and from mother to child. It is important to distinguish persons who are infected with the virus but show no symptoms (HIV antibody positive) from those who have developed symptoms of AIDS. AIDS affects both developing and industrialised countries. However, economic difficulties and weaker health care infrastructure make it difficult for developing countries to mount effective prevention and control programmes for AIDS.

According to UNAIDS by the end of the year 2002 there were:

- 3.1 million deaths due to HIV/AIDS in 2002 – of which 500,000 were children,
- 42 million people living with HIV/AIDS,
- 5.1 million new HIV infections over the whole of the year 2002 – more than 95% of these were in developing countries, over half of the infected adults were under 25 years old.

The new health problems

Developing countries are taking up many health problems of industrialised countries.

Part of the reason for this shift can be explained simply by the fact that, as conditions improve, people are living longer and there are more chronic diseases such as heart disease and cancers. However, other reasons are the dramatic social changes taking place in developing countries:

- increased numbers of elderly persons in the population requiring care and support;
- expansion of cities and urban living resulting in greater mobility, poor housing, separation of families and removal of traditional systems of support;
- increased industrialisation resulting in pollution and occupational diseases including accidents, exposure to harmful dust, chemicals and noise;
- more motor cars and traffic leading to an increase in deaths from more road traffic accidents;
- sexually transmitted diseases and AIDS encouraged by changing patterns of sexual behaviour, breaking up of family structures, growth of sex tourism;
- changes in diet especially sugar, fat and salt resulting in increase in dental decay, obesity, heart disease, hypertension, diabetes, cancer of the bowel, appendicitis – the 'diseases of westernisation'. WHO estimates that at least half of all deaths from cardiovascular diseases can be prevented;
- greater availability of addictive substances including tobacco, alcohol and drugs;
- conflicts of commercial interests and health – the damage done by advertising and promotion of tobacco, baby milk, cigarettes and inappropriate medicines;
- globalisation – the increasing interdependence of the economies in different parts of the world in trade and finance and the reduction in the power of individual countries.

Tobacco-induced diseases

Worldwide over one billion people now smoke – averaging over ten cigarettes a day. Many traditional forms of tobacco are smoked, such as the bidi leaf cigarettes in India. More and more people are switching to cigarettes, which account for about 75% of all tobacco consumed.

Tobacco affects health in many ways – through the nicotine, tar and the effect of the carbon monoxide in the smoke on the body function. The health risks of tobacco include: greater likelihood of suffering from diseases including lung cancer, heart disease and respiratory disorders. Families, friends and work colleagues of smokers can be harmed through *passive smoking* – the harmful effects of cigarette smoke breathed in by non-smokers.

Cigarette sales in developing countries are growing faster than other countries. About 4 million people die every year from tobacco-related diseases. If current trends continue WHO estimate that the toll will rise to 10 million every year by 2030. Tobacco is becoming a greater cause of death and disability than any other single disease. Young people in particular are taking up the habit. About 20% of schoolchildren in developing countries are already regular smokers. Some 250 million children and teenagers alive today will eventually die as a result of their tobacco habit and 70% of them will be in developing countries.

- In Bangladesh the money spent on just five cigarettes a day could pay for one-quarter of a child's daily food needs.
- The firewood used in curing tobacco worldwide is equivalent to 2.8 million hectares of land each year.
- 0.3% of the world's farming land is used for tobacco – enough to feed 10–12 million people if the same land were used for grain.

Violence

Until recently this important cause of disability and death had been neglected by health services. In the year 2000 an estimated 1.6 million people worldwide lost their lives to violence. Around half of those deaths were suicides, and

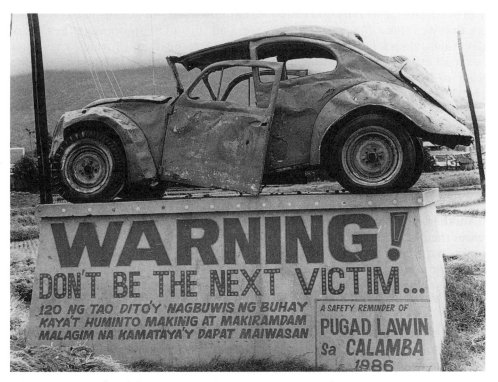

Fig. 1.3   Social changes in the developing countries are leading to new health problems such as traffic accidents

nearly one-third were homicides. The true extent of the problem of violence is much greater as most cases of violence result in injury, disability and problems of mental health. The causes are far ranging and include domestic violence against women, rape and child abuse. In 1996 the World Health Assembly adopted a resolution declaring violence a leading wordwide public health problem.

Influences on health

In order to decide what actions are needed to prevent disease and promote health we need to be able to identify influences on health. In particular, we need to be able to distinguish those causes about which very little can be done from others that we *can* change. One factor we cannot change is the genes we have acquired through inheritance from our parents. For example, a person born with the genetic disorder sickle-cell anaemia has the disease for life and should receive counselling to help them to cope with it. The influences of climate, geography and genetic inheritance that we cannot change are sometimes called non-behavioural influences.

But many causes of disease can be changed. To prevent disease we must concentrate on those causes that we can change and these are the factors to which that we must devote our attentions.

There are other ways of looking at influences. Later in this chapter you will see how it is possible to consider the *level of influence* – whether the factors that influence health are under the individual's control or operate at the family, community, district, national or international level. Another approach is to separate out those influences that are *cultural*.

An approach that I have found useful is the *Health Field Model* used by the Canadian Government in their influential policy document 'The Health of the Canadians'. As a practical model, it separates the influences into four interrelated areas: those due to human biology or genetics, behaviour or 'life style'; those that can be influenced by improved health-care systems; and those that are determined by the environment (see Figure 1.4).

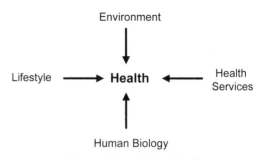

Fig. 1.4   Health Field Model and influences on health

Human biology

The recent progress of the Human Genome Project in mapping human chromosomes represents a stunning achievement for medical science. It is clear that our susceptibility to many diseases is heavily dependent on our genetic inheritance. While our genetics shapes our health, the relationship is not a simple one. A person's health status is a result of an interaction of genetics, environment, exposure to infective agents and the lifestyle they lead. Some of the harmful effects of genetic diseases can be moderated through appropriate health services. Genetic counselling provides a mechanism for us to obtain greater awareness of how we can influence of our genetic inheritance through choice of partner and through changes in diet and lifestyle. Health services are setting up pre-natal testing for genetic abnormalities although this raises many difficult ethical issues.

Environment

According to WHO, almost one third of the global burden of disease can be attributed to environmental risk factors. The environment, especially climate, has an important influence on our health. Disease, food production and access to drinking water are influenced by temperature, rainfall, soil conditions and vegetation. Diseases such as diarrhoea and malaria have a higher incidence in the rainy season. Deserts, forests, swamps and coastal regions will all affect health of their communities.

Although the environment has a profound effect on health, its effects are linked to other factors, especially the behaviours and actions of people. For example building of dams, irrigation projects, cutting of forests, overgrazing of land by animals, use of pesticides, factory pollution and wars can all affect the environment and health. In recent years there has been serious concern about the impact on global warming because of release of greenhouse gases such as carbon dioxide from factories, motor cars, power stations and other human activities. Global warming is already leading to changes in climate and increased level of disease and it has been difficult to get governments to take action to reduce the emissions of greenhouse gases.

Even so-called 'natural' disasters such as earthquakes, volcanic eruptions, hurricanes and cyclones raise some important questions about human behaviour and social forces. What conditions make people live in disaster-prone areas? Why can't the poor afford to build houses strong enough to resist earthquakes?

The contribution of health services to health

In recent years more and more people are asking the question: *do health services make people healthy?* In most countries, too much emphasis is put on treatment rather than prevention, urban rather than rural health and meeting health needs of the richer sections of the community rather than the poor.

The introduction of the concept of *Primary Health Care* by the World Health Assembly in the city of Alma Ata in 1978 was a direct result of the failure of curative hospital-based systems of health care. It was realised that most of the important health problems in the world can be dealt with by a combination of decentralised basic health care and prevention. The *Alma Ata Declaration* went on to say:

> Primary health care is essential health care based on practical, scientifically sound and socially acceptable methods and technology made universally accessible to individuals and families in the community through their full participation and at a cost that the community and country can afford to maintain at every stage of their development in the spirit of self-reliance and self-determination.

The full text of the Alma Ata Declaration is a remarkable document that emphasised the importance of preventive measures including provision of food, housing, water, sanitation and health education. It also clearly stated that improvement of health cannot be separated from discussions about social concerns such as poverty and social justice.

The idea of primary health care does not ignore the significant role that medicine can make to improvement of health through the provision of treatment, immunisation and screening. However, health services should be *appropriate* – effective, affordable and acceptable to the communities. When you are considering a health issue such as a cholera outbreak, diarrhoea, lung cancer or maternal health there are some fundamental questions that you should ask to decide what role, if any, health services can play:

- How good is our current understanding about the health topic? Can it be prevented? Is there a vaccine available? Can we screen people at risk or at early stages of the disease?
- What, if any, health services are necessary for prevention?
- How effective are home remedies and traditional medicines?
- Can it be cured? Are drugs available?
- If the disease cannot be cured, what can be done to make the condition of the patient as comfortable as possible?
- What kinds of health services are needed for treatment and care at lowest cost to the community?

Human behaviour

Most health issues cannot be dealt with by drugs and treatment alone. The promotion of health and prevention of disease will usually involve some changes in lifestyles or human behaviour. There can be confusion over terms used.

- The words **actions**, **practices** and **behaviours** are different words for the same thing.
- *Lifestyle* refers to the collection of behaviours that makes up a person's way of life – including diet, clothing, family life, housing and work.

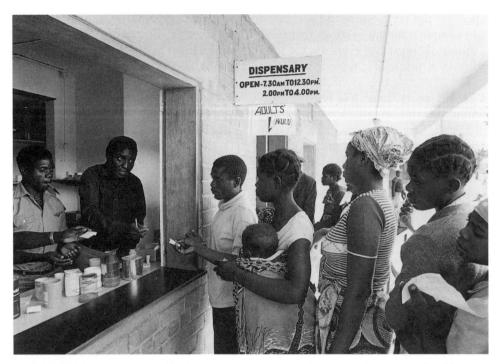

Fig.1.5   Health services on their own cannot prevent disease and promote health

- *Customs* are behaviours that many people share.
- *Traditions* are behaviours that have been carried out for a long time and handed down from parents to children.

Here are listed some of the many kinds of behaviours that have an influence on health, and the 13 key behaviours for improvement of child health that UNICEF, WHO and UNESCO identified in their initiative *Facts for Life*.

Examples of behaviours promoting health and preventing disease

Health behaviours: actions that healthy people undertake to keep themselves or others healthy and prevent disease, e.g. exercise, good nutrition, breastfeeding, weaning, latrines, child-spacing, hygiene practices, tooth-brushing, taking anti-malaria drugs; reduction of health-damaging behaviours such as smoking, bottle-feeding, excessive alcohol consumption and accidents. These behaviours may be based on decisions or are done regularly and have become habits – or routines.

Utilisation behaviours: utilisation of health services such as antenatal, child health, immunisation, family planning and screening programmes.

Illness behaviours: recognition of early symptoms and prompt self-referral for treatment such as oral rehydration and leprosy.

Compliance behaviours: following of course of prescribed drugs such as for tuberculosis.

Rehabilitation behaviours: what people need to do after a serious illness to prevent further disability.

Community action: actions by individuals and groups to change and improve their surroundings.

The essential messages from *Facts of Life*

1. The health of both women and children can be significantly improved when births are spaced at least 2 years apart, when pregnancy is avoided before age 18 and after age 35, and when a woman has no more than four pregnancies in total.

2. All pregnant women should visit a health worker for prenatal care, and all births should be assisted by a skilled birth attendant. All pregnant women and their families need to know the warning signs of problems during pregnancy and have plans for obtaining immediate skilled help if problems arise.

3. Children learn from the moment of birth. They grow and learn fastest when they receive attention, affection and stimulation, in addition to good nutrition and proper health care. Encouraging children to observe and to express themselves, to play and explore, helps them learn and develop socially, physically and intellectually.

4. Breast milk *alone* is the only food and drink an infant needs for the first 6 months. After 6 months, infants need other foods in addition to breast milk.

5. Poor nutrition during the mother's pregnancy or during the child's first 2 years can slow a child's mental and physical development for life. From birth to age two, children should be weighed every month. If a young child does not gain weight over a 2-month period, something is wrong.

6. Every child needs a series of immunisations during the first year of life to protect against diseases that can cause poor growth, disability or death. Every woman of childbearing age needs to be protected against tetanus. Even if the woman was immunised earlier, she needs to check with a health worker.

7. A child with diarrhoea needs to drink plenty of the right liquids – breast milk, fruit juice or oral rehydration solution (ORS). If the diarrhoea is bloody or frequent and watery, the child is in danger and should be taken to a health centre for immediate treatment.

8. Most children with coughs or colds will get better on their own. But if a child with a cough is breathing rapidly or with difficulty, the child is in danger and needs to be taken to a health centre for immediate treatment.

9. Many illnesses can be prevented by good hygiene practices – using clean toilets or latrines, washing hands with soap and water or ash and water after defecating and before handling food, using water from a safe source, and keeping food and water clean.

10. Malaria, which is transmitted through mosquito bites, can be fatal. Wherever malaria is common, mosquito nets treated with a recommended insecticide should be used, any child with a fever should be examined by a trained health worker, and pregnant women should take antimalarial tablets recommended by a health worker.

11. AIDS is a fatal but preventable disease. HIV, the virus that causes AIDS, spreads through unprotected sex (intercourse without a condom), transfusions of unscreened blood, contaminated needles and syringes (most often those used for injecting drugs), and from an infected woman to her child during pregnancy, childbirth or breast-feeding. It is essential for everyone to know about HIV/AIDS and how to prevent it. The risk of infection through the primary sexual route can be reduced by practising safer sex. Women who are or could be infected with HIV should consult a qualified health worker for information, counselling and testing to protect their health and reduce the risk of infecting their infants.

12. Many serious accidents can be prevented if parents or caretakers watch young children carefully and keep their environment safe.

13. In disaster or emergency situations, children should receive essential health care, including measles vaccination and micronutrient supplementation. In stressful situations, it is always preferable for children to be cared for by their parents or other familiar adults. Breastfeeding is particularly important at this time.

Inequalities in health

The Health Field Model helps us to understand why some people enjoy better health than others. Each of us has a different set of genes that determine the characteristics we inherit from our parents. However, most of the differences in health that exist cannot be explained by genetic differences. They are a result of differences in the living conditions and communities in which a person grows up, especially inequalities in:

- income, purchasing power and food consumption;
- housing and living conditions;
- educational opportunities;
- geography and place of residence, including rural versus urban, and exposure to environmental hazards such as flooding, earthquakes and hurricanes;
- access to health services;
- gender – different opportunities, expectations and roles of men and women.

Inequalities in health pose a challenge to all of us who are working to improve the health of communities. Facing up to this challenge involves redirecting services to meet the needs of those with the worst health and directly tackling the root causes of inequalities.

The role of human behaviour in prevention of disease

There are three levels of prevention (see Figure 1.6).

Primary prevention

The purpose of primary prevention is to keep healthy people healthy and prevent them getting disease. It involves public health measures such as immunisation, improved water supply, vector control and fluoridation, preventive services such as family planning, the promotion of health behaviours and the discouraging of health-damaging behaviours.

Secondary prevention

Secondary prevention is the name given to interventions at the early stage of a problem before it becomes serious. It is important to ensure that the community can recognise early signs of disease and go for treatment before the disease becomes serious. Health problems such as leprosy and tuberculosis can be cured if the disease is caught at an early stage. The actions people take before consulting a health care worker including recognition of symptoms, taking home remedies ('self-medication'), consulting family and healers are called *illness behaviours* and are shown below in Figure 1.7.

Screening is the name given to the process of surveying a community with tests to detect diseases at an early stage before people feel symptoms. A good example of this is the cervical smear test, which detects unusual 'pre-cancerous' cells in a woman's cervix before they develop into cancer. Another example of screening is growth monitoring of young children. It is not easy to tell just by looking at a child if he or she is malnourished. However, if the child is regularly weighed and the weights are plotted on a growth chart, you can see from the chart if there is a slowing-down of growth. Advice can then be given to the parents to prevent the child becoming malnourished. Although screening is carried out by health services, educational programmes are still needed to encourage people to come forward for screening.

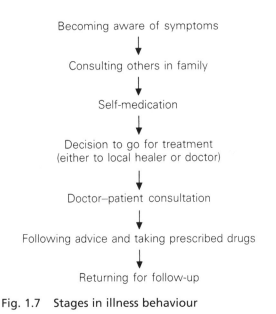

Fig. 1.7   Stages in illness behaviour

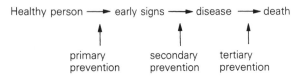

Fig. 1.6   Levels of prevention of disease

Tertiary prevention

It is better to prevent disease. But people will still get sick and need treatment. Even at this stage actions and behaviours of the patient are essential to getting well again. Tertiary prevention overlaps with secondary prevention and includes behaviours that are involved in treatment and rehabilitation.

Recovery from treatment and operations may involve some rehabilitation programmes. For example after a period in bed a person may need physiotherapy and exercise to recover full strength. Help is needed for a person to adjust to artificial limbs or using a wheelchair. The rehabilitation process can involve meeting both a person's physical and psychological needs.

An important part of tertiary prevention is to ensure patients *follow treatment procedures*: if patients are prescribed medicines, it is essential that they take them correctly. The health worker must explain when to take them, for how long and what to do if there are any side effects.

Tuberculosis is a good example of the importance of following treatment procedures. The drugs for treatment of tuberculosis are effective but it is important to take a complete course of treatment. People often mistakenly believe that they are cured once they feel better, stop taking the drugs and experience a relapse of tuberculosis. The Directly Observed Treatment Shortcourse (DOTS) approach puts special emphasis on ensuring that a full course is completed. Doctors may prescribe unnecessary drugs and the patients sometimes insist on being given a medicine. For example, many children with diarrhoea are prescribed antibiotics, which are not effective against most childhood diarrhoea and delay the life-saving oral rehydration. The overuse of medicine can be an expensive drain on the budget of the family and the health services, and it also encourages the development of antibiotic-resistant bacteria. Control of commercial drug advertising, training of doctors and education of the public are all important factors in the reduction of unnecessary prescribing of drugs.

However, the real danger of unnecessary use of medicines is not the one of cost, but encouragement of the belief that achievement of health lies only in medicines. It draws attention away from the need for actions by governments and individuals to improve living conditions and encourage health-promoting behaviours.

Behavioural diagnosis

The term behavioural diagnosis is used to describe the process by which we look at the causes of the health problems and find out whether human behaviour is involved – either in prevention or treatment. In the behavioural diagnosis we list all the actions that the community should carry out for primary, secondary and tertiary prevention of the disease. It is the behaviours of the persons *themselves* in the community that are identified. Later in the planning stage you will have to consider what determines these behaviours; especially the role of social and economic factors such as poverty, inequalities, inappropriate health services and government policies.

The key messages in 'Facts for Life' are an example of the behavioural diagnosis applied to a general health topic – child health. We can also apply the concept of behavioural diagnosis to general programme areas such as water and sanitation. The role of health education and communication support in promoting uptake of water and sanitation technologies and achieving health benefits is shown in the list.

Behavioural diagnoses of water and sanitation programmes

- community participation in the installation of improved water supply;
- use and maintenance of improved water supplies including avoidance of unimproved sources, clean collection and storage of water in the home;
- building of latrines and upgrading of unimproved latrines to improved latrines;
- correct use of latrines, especially by groups such as children;
- maintaining the new improved latrines;
- hygiene practices especially washing of hands with soap after use of latrines and before preparation of food and eating; washing of faces; clean storage of food and utensils; personal hygiene, washing of children and babies; washing of clothing; disposal of dirty water from washing etc.

Our changing knowledge

There are many examples where health educators have wasted time and effort persuading people to adopt practices that we later found were not relevant. For example, in the 1980s many health workers mistakenly encouraged mothers to give high protein foods to children to prevent the form of malnutrition called kwashiorkor. We now know that lack of protein foods in the diet is not a direct cause of kwashiorkor and nutritionists emphasise adding oils/fats to weaning diets to enrich the energy content.

Although our understanding of health and disease is improving, many fieldworkers are still using out-of-date and inaccurate information in their health education. Even the so-called 'experts' do not always agree. The public can get very confused with conflicting messages and do not know which to follow. It is not surprising that they often become impatient and ignore us!

But, as knowledge improves, you should continually expect changes in the future. A good way for you to keep up with new developments is to put yourself on the mailing list of the free newsletters produced by international agencies (see Appendix). The growth of the Internet has provided new opportunities for the increasing numbers of persons with access to computers.

The need to understand human behaviour

It is a common complaint that the community ignore advice and continue to practise health damaging behaviours even if they know that they are harmful. It is easy to condemn the community and put the blame on traditional beliefs or backwardness. The real reason for failure, however, is often that the health promotion doesn't take into account the underlying influences on health, contains irrelevant information, promotes unrealistic changes, is directed at the wrong people and uses inappropriate methods. So, to promote health, it is important to determine the factors that underlie a person's decision to perform or not perform a behaviour.

Human behaviour plays an important role in the prevention, control, treatment and rehabilitation processes of most health problems. However, Table 1.1 shows that the influences on a person's behaviour may be outside the individual at the family, community, district, national and even international level.

Some problems, such as lack of water are too big to be tackled by individual families. The whole community must act together to deal with these. So in looking at the influences on a behaviour we may decide that the change must take place at the level of the whole community. Our understanding of behaviour may show that there are many influences outside the individual's control that are actually *damaging* health. These outside influences could include advertising health-damaging products such as cigarettes or baby foods, government policies such as promoting tobacco cultivation or location of health services, poverty and unemployment. *Victim-blaming is the name given to the process when poorly planned health education directs itself at changing the individual and ignores the factors outside the individual that influence behaviour.*

Health promotion

Many feel that too much effort has been placed on programmes aimed at individuals. They have pointed to the importance of working with communities to influence economic and political factors at the community or national level. They have stressed the need to persuade governments to pass health-promoting laws such as control of advertising of tobacco and baby foods, and supporting the expansion of primary health care programmes and agricultural development. Another concern that was voiced was the need to address inequalities in health, which involves actions beyond the traditional role of health services.

The term *health promotion* is increasingly being used to draw attention to the need for both educational and political action to improve health – especially of disadvantaged groups. At a meeting in Canada in 1986, the

Table 1.1 Influences on health at different levels

Individual	Family	Community	National	International
Beliefs, values and attitudes of individual person only	Beliefs, values and attitudes held at family level – the family culture	Beliefs, values and attitudes held at community level – community culture	Beliefs, values and attitudes shared by whole nation – national culture	Globalisation of cultures, ideas
Personal experience	Family experiences	Community experiences	Mass media advertising and marketing by commercial companies	Multinational companies – advertising and promotion of products
Susceptibility to pressure from family and community	Patterns of influence and decision-making in the family	Influence of community leaders, elders and opinion leaders	National level institutions, e.g. Professional bodies	International UN Agencies (WHO, World Bank, UNICEF, IMF etc.)
Knowledge, skills and education	Knowledge, skills and education of family members	Quantity, quality and appropriateness of local services: health, education, sanitation, agriculture	Government policies on health, education, income, water, gender rights etc.	International pressure groups
Genetic endowment	Economic situation of family	Socio-economic situation of family	Socio-economic situation of country	Global economic situation
Economic situation of individual				

Ottawa Charter on Health Promotion was drawn up. This conference mainly focused on the needs in industrialised countries, but also took into account similar concerns in other regions. The Charter emphasised that promoting health is more than just providing health services. Peace, housing, education, food, income, a sustainable environment, social justice and equity are all necessary for achievement of health. It calls for people to act as *advocates* for health through the addressing of political, economic, social, cultural, environmental, behavioural and biological factors.

Ethics of health promotion and behaviour change

Most health promotion programmes seek to influence families, the community and decision makers to make changes, either in their own lives, or in policies that affect other people's health. This raises important questions about the ethics of interventions. Look at the questions below. How you would answer them?

- Is it right for health promoters to persuade or pass laws to influence people to change their behaviour?
- Under what conditions do you think it might be justified to try to make someone do something that they do not want to do?
- When do you think it is better to leave the persons themselves to make the decision as to the behaviour change? Can people living in a state of poverty and oppression make decisions and control their own lives? How can health promoters encourage this process?

These questions pose important *ethical* issues. Some people argue that individuals should have the right to do what they want to do and we should not interfere. This is a common response when we try to persuade smokers to give up.

But should a person have the freedom to choose, if their actions may also harm others?

Extracts from the Ottawa Charter on Health Promotion

'Health promotion is the process of enabling people to increase control over, and to improve, their health. To reach a state of complete physical, mental and social well-being, an individual or group must be able to identify and to realise aspirations, to satisfy needs, and to change or cope with the environment. Health is, therefore, seen as a resource for everyday life, not the objective of living. Health is a positive concept emphasising social and personal resources, as well as physical capacities. Therefore, health promotion is not just the responsibility of the health sector, but goes beyond healthy lifestyles to well-being.'

HEALTH PROMOTION ACTION MEANS:

Building Healthy Public Policy Health promotion goes beyond health care. It puts health on the agenda of policy makers in all sectors and at all levels. It directs policy makers to be aware of the health consequences of their decisions and accept their responsibilities for health.

Health promotion policy combines diverse but complementary approaches including legislation, fiscal measures, taxation and organisational change. It is coordinated action that leads to health, income and social policies that foster greater equity. Joint action contributes to ensuring safer and healthier goods and services, healthier public services, and cleaner, more enjoyable environments.

Health promotion policy requires the identification of obstacles to the adoption of healthy public policies in non-health sectors, and ways of removing them. The aim must be to make the healthier choice the easier choice.

Creating Supportive Environments Health promotion generates living and working conditions that are safe, stimulating, satisfying and enjoyable. Systematic assessment of the health impact of a rapidly changing environment – particularly in areas of technology, work, energy production and urbanisation – is essential and must be followed by action to ensure positive benefit to the health of the public. The protection of the natural and built environments and the conservation of natural resources must be addressed in any health promotion strategy.

Strengthening Community Action At the heart of this process is the empowerment of communities, their ownership and control of their own endeavours and destinies. Community development draws on existing human and material resources in the community to enhance self-help and social support, and to develop flexible systems for strengthening public participation and direction of health matters.

Developing Personal Skills Health promotion supports personal and social development through providing information, education for health and enhancing life skills. By so doing, it increases the options available to people to exercise more control over their health and environment, and to make choices conducive to health. Enabling people to learn throughout life, to prepare themselves for all of its stages and to cope with chronic illness and injuries is essential. This has to be facilitated in school, home, work and community settings. Action is required through educational, professional, commercial and voluntary bodies, and within the institutions themselves.

Reorienting Health Services The responsibility for health promotion in health services is shared among individuals, community groups, health professionals, health service institutions and governments. They must work together towards a health care system that contributes to the pursuit of health. Reorienting health services also requires stronger attention to health research as well as changes in professional education and training. This must lead to a change of attitude and organisation of health services, which refocuses on the total needs of the individual as a whole person.

For example a person who smokes is not only damaging his or her own health but also others who breathe in the smoke – for example their children. Someone who drinks alcohol while driving can endanger other people's lives. A food handler has a responsibility to practise good hygiene to preserve the health of those who consume their food. Public health often involves restricting the behaviour of individuals for the good of the community. However, the decisions on what should be changed are not only medical ones –

but involve social, religious and moral considerations.

Some people argue that the community should be left to make their own decisions. However the community may have an incomplete understanding of health and diseases: they may not be aware of the existence of innovations such as immunisation, oral rehydration therapy or improved pit-latrines. Failure to tell the community about these life-saving new practices might also be considered unethical.

You will have to apply two further ethical conditions before deciding to intervene. The first is that you have made certain that the proposed intervention will not harm the intended beneficiaries, and the second is that that it will lead to improvements in their health.

Evidence-based practice

In recent years increased importance has been placed on making decisions based on evidence. This means using methods that have been shown to be effective through a systematic process of research and evaluation. While most people would agree with the idea that our efforts should be based on what works, in practice this is not always easy. People can disagree over what should be considered as evidence and how to measure effectiveness. Some activities, especially using community participation, can be difficult to evaluate. It is not always easy to find out details of programmes that have been evaluated. In writing this book I have emphasised evidence-based methods and provided case studies of programmes taken from the Leeds Health Education Database of evaluated interventions from developing countries. In the final chapter of this book you will find more information on evaluation and the issues involved in measuring impact and judging effectiveness.

Health promotion interventions and HESIAD

An effective intervention will usually have to address three key areas of activity, which can easily be remembered using the abbreviation HESIAD – Health Education, Service Improvement and Advocacy – see Figure 1.8.

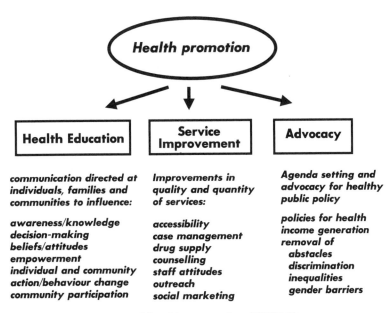

Fig. 1.8   Components of health promotion (HESIAD)

Health education

Information and education provide the informed base for making choices. They are necessary and core components of health promotion, which aims at **increasing knowledge and disseminating information** related to health. This should include: the public's perceptions and experiences of health and how it might be sought; knowledge from epidemiology, social and other sciences on the patterns of health and disease and factors affecting them; and descriptions of the 'total' environment in which health and health choices are shaped.

(WHO Policy statement on Health Promotion)

Health education is one of the most important components of health promotion and involves activities directed at individuals, families and communities for:

- motivation to adopt health-promoting behaviours;
- helping people to make decisions about their health and acquire the necessary confidence and skills to put their decisions into practice.

The American health educator Lawrence Green defines health education as: 'any combination of learning opportunities designed to facilitate voluntary adaptation of behaviour which will improve or maintain health'. The use of the word voluntary is significant for ethical reasons. It implies that health educators should not force people to do what they do not want to do. Instead our efforts should help people to make decisions and choices for themselves.

Helen Ross and Paul Mico have provided another useful definition of health education: 'A process with intellectual, psychological and social dimensions relating to activities that increase the abilities of people to make informed decisions affecting their personal family and community well-being. This process, based on scientific principles, facilitates learning and behavioural change in both health personnel and consumers, including children and youth.' The term health education will be used throughout this book to cover health education and broadly similar activities carried out under different names. Some alternative terms in the list are equivalent to health education, others are based on narrower approaches and assumptions.

Various terms used for communication and health education activities

Information, education and communication (IEC) is a term originally from family planning and more recently AIDS control programmes in developing countries. It is increasingly being used as a general term for communication activities to promote health.

Behaviour change communication is a term that has recently been introduced to describe activities directed at promoting healthy behaviours in communities.

Health communication is a term widely used in USA and promoted by the Communication Initiative Internet web site.

Communication support is a term for describing support programmes for introduction of water, sanitation and hygiene education. Heili Perret has defined communication support as 'Information, motivation and education activities which are specifically designed to encourage the participation of intended beneficiaries in a project and to improve the project's impact on development.'

Social marketing involves the application of commercial marketing and advertising approaches to health and has been used for promotion of condoms, oral rehydration solution and mosquito nets.

Social mobilisation is a term now popular with UNICEF to describe a campaign approach combining mass media and working with community groups and organisations.

Extension comes originally from the agricultural extension approach of promoting change through demonstrations, working with opinion leaders and community-based educational activities.

Nutrition education is education directed at the promotion of nutrition and covers choice of food, food preparation and storage.

Population education includes education on family planning; *family life education* is another related term for education of young people in a range of topics that include family planning, child rearing and child care and responsible parenthood.

Patient education is a term for education in hospital and clinic settings linked to following of treatment procedures, medication, home care, rehabilitation procedures.

Other 'education' activities. Antenatal education, AIDS education, dental health education, mental health education are all specialised areas of health education.

Service improvement

Improvements in service delivery can include any of the following:

*   *Improvements in the content of the service,* e.g. improved case management, counselling, patient education, outreach to communities, schools and workplace.
*   *Improvements in the accessibility of the service,* e.g. timing, location and the introduction of home and community visits.
*   *Improvements in the acceptability of services,* e.g. enforcement of confidentiality, use of women field staff, use of lay field staff, involvement of persons from the target community.

The changes required will depend on the topic area and local needs. The main actions needed to improve services usually involve setting up of guidelines, reorientation of staff roles and training. For further information on design of training programmes see Chapter 4 and on interpersonal skills and patient education see Chapter 5.

Advocacy

Advocacy involves activities directed at policy-makers to influence laws and policies concerning the allocation of resources, priorities for expenditure, direction of services and enforcement of laws. The term agenda setting is used for activities designed to raise the profile of neglected issues, e.g. provision for the elderly or the need for legal reform. It is not easy to influence issues such as the status of women, discriminatory laws, poverty and prejudice. Many of them are *structural*, i.e. determined at the regional, national and even international level, and not easy to change by activities at the community level. There may also be opposition to change from influential vested interests, such as rich and powerful people, commercial companies and foreign countries. Because of the difficulties and controversial nature of advocacy, many interventions leave this out. However, advocacy may be a vital and necessary part of your activities if your programme is to have an impact.

The advocacy component of an intervention will usually consist of a mixture of *short-term* and *long-term* activities.

*   *Short term activities* are those that are achievable during the time scale of the intervention (usually 3–5 years) and that will have some impact on improving the situation. These might include income-generating activities, subsidies on essential supplies, e.g. condoms/medicines, changes in the interpretation/enforcement of laws by the police and the initiation of debate on the need to change laws.
*   *Long-term activities* are those that usually take more than 5 years to accomplish. These consist of major legal changes and shifts in policy.

Activities for achieving short- and long-term changes involve encouragement of debate and discussion – through mass media, seminars and meetings with politicians, community leaders and the general public.

Some public health officials have put forward the view that health education is not necessary and that improvements in health can be achieved by political change and policy alone. An example given in support of this view is that of wearing of seatbelts in cars, which was only widely practised in the United Kingdom once laws were passed. However, just passing a law on its own is not usually enough to ensure full compliance and health benefits. For example in an urban housing scheme in Lesotho permission was only given to build a house if it had a latrine. While people complied with the law and built latrines, some people were not convinced of their value and were using them as storehouses.

Governments may be reluctant to pass laws unless there is popular support. Health education directed at communities can be needed to create a climate of public opinion that will support a change in law. Even after a law is passed, health education is needed to ensure full understanding of the importance of compliance.

Guidelines on the use of media to influence policy are provided in Chapter 8 and a summary of advocacy methods for influencing policy is given in Chapter 10.

Communication in health promotion

In its simplest form, communication involves exchanges of information between people. All three components of health promotion – health education, service improvement and advocacy involve communication in some form or other in order to achieve the following:

- make dialogue with communities, including minorities, disadvantaged groups to promote health empowerment, influence beliefs and develop skills;
- ensure that the public gives support to government health-promoting policies;
- communicate new laws and policies to the public;
- raise public awareness of issues in order to mobilise community participation;
- develop community action on health issues;
- convince the public of the need for service improvements and additional resources;
- train staff in new skills;
- manage, supervise and support improved services;
- influence decision-makers to adopt health-promoting policies and laws;
- raise awareness among decision-makers of issues of poverty, human rights, equity and environmental issues;
- encourage different services to work together to tackle problems in the community.

Chapter 3 discusses the different ways that communication can happen and the psychological processes involved.

What approach to use?

Even if the main aim of health education is to influence behaviour, there is a range of possible approaches that include:

- The *persuasion approach* – the deliberate attempt to influence the other person to do what we want them to do (often called the 'directive' approach, or when done forcefully it is called coercion).
- The *health empowerment approach* – giving people information, problem-solving and decision-making skills to make *informed decisions* and building confidence and power to put those decisions into practice.

One educationalist who has had a profound influence is Paulo Freire. He was deeply critical of formal 'didactic' approaches to education where the teacher was seen to be the expert passing knowledge to the pupils. In his literacy work among the peasants of Northeast Brazil, he pioneered an alternative approach to education called 'conscientisation' also called consciousness raising. His methods aimed to develop critical awareness, raising of consciousness and stimulating people to think how they can change their environment.

Many health educators feel that, instead of using persuasion and coercion, it is better to work with communities to develop their problem-solving skills and provide the information to help them make *informed choices*. A key to this is the concept of *health literacy* – defined by Don Nutbeam as 'the cognitive and social skills which determine the motivation and abilities of individuals to gain access to, understand and use information in ways to promote and maintain good health.' On its own health literacy is not enough, people need to have *self-efficacy* – a term introduced by the American psychologist Alfred Bandura to describe a person's beliefs and confidence that he or she has the power and ability to change their surroundings. The relationship between these concepts can be summarised as:

Health Empowerment = Self-efficacy + Health Literacy

More information on self-efficacy is provided in the discussion on Social Learning Theory in Chapter 2, and the ideas of Paulo Freire and the methods for promoting empowerment are explored in Chapter 6.

Persuasion approaches seek to achieve changes in specific behaviours. The health empowerment approach looks to promote a longer-term change in the way individuals and communities look at the world in which they live. Persuasion approaches have been applied in situations where communities have the resources to act and change their situation and there is a readily identifiable and effective solution to the problem.

The health empowerment approach is often used in situations when there is no clear desired outcome and the individual and community need to make the choice that is best for them, e.g. in counselling on sensitive issues such as family planning and reduction of risk for HIV/AIDS. Empowerment approaches have also been used when individuals and communities lack power, are oppressed and living in poverty and exploitation. Chapter 2 will explain how some behaviours are more complex to change than others and may require health empowerment methods. With some people a decision on whether to use a persuasion approach or an empowerment approach is one of personal belief, ideology and philosophy. With others it is a question of choosing the right approach to match the situation and time available.

Should you focus on specific diseases or promote health?

You will need to decide whether to focus on prevention of particular diseases, e.g. AIDS, diarrhoea, or whether to take a broader approach. The advantage of taking a single-disease approach is that it is often easier to mobilise the public, other fieldworkers and potential sponsors on a single issue. However many prefer the broader approach because they feel that it is better to emphasise health and a healthy lifestyle rather than disease. In health care planning, the name given to the approach that focuses on individual diseases is 'vertical' planning whereas the alternative of taking a broader health-focused approach is 'horizontal'.

Who should the education be directed at?

An individual's behaviour is extremely important for his or her health. But it is not always the individual who makes the decisions and should be the 'target group'. We often find that a person's behaviour is influenced by other persons in the family and community and these social pressures are examined further in the next chapter. Communications should be directed at the persons who make the key decisions in the family and community – the 'gatekeepers'.

Even when you have decided on a particular 'target group' you will need to consider at what point in that person's life is the best time to reach them. We can think of the human life cycle, or *health career*, as a series of stages from the young child to the school-aged child to the adult and the elderly person (Figure 1.9). In the educational diagnosis we must decide at what stage to carry out our health education. A well-planned programme will include educational activities directed at a range of different age groups.

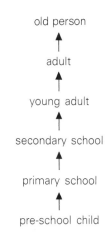

Fig. 1.9 A 'Health Career'. At what stage in the human life cycle to intervene?

At what level should the intervention take place?

You could operate your communication activities at range of levels: individual, family, community, district, region, national and international. For example you could work with individuals using one-to-one education, you could spend time with the family, mobilise community participation or act at a national level to influence policy.

How you choose the level to operate at will depend on the problems you are facing, the special advantages to be gained from each level and the resources and opportunities that are available to you. Your analysis of the influences on behaviour (see Table 1.1) might have told you that the important influences that you have to change are at one level, e.g. at the national level. However, if you are based in a local community you may not be able to work at the national level.

What channel or setting can you work through?

You will have to decide on the best way of reaching your intended audience – home, community, clinics, school, workplace, markets, public places, bars or clubs? For example, women of childbearing age can often be reached through child health services, adult men could be reached through the workplace and children through schools. Mass media such as radio would be suitable for reaching the general population, whereas messages for specific groups are best communicated through face-to-face communication.

The 'settings' approach has now been widely adopted in health promotion. This involves identifying relevant settings that can be used to improve the health of those who use the setting and the community. In some case these settings have formed the basis of international movements, e.g. the Healthy Cities Programme, the Health Promoting Schools, and the Health Promoting Hospital. In these movements, targets have been agreed of what a particular city, hospital or school needs to achieve to qualify for membership of the movement. Experiences are shared by members through networks of newsletters and conferences.

Decisions are also needed as to *who* will implement the programme. Are there people, such as teachers, youth leaders, employers, politicians, musicians, who you can involve in educational activities? A powerful approach is to use people from the same background as the people you are trying to reach – a method called peer education. Health education and health promotion are part of the work of a wide range of persons in health, education, social and other services who might be mobilised to support your activities. You might decide to work through non-governmental agencies such as Red Cross, Red Crescent, planned parenthood associations, churches, boy scouts or self-help and community-based groups. As part of primary health care activities, many countries have mobilised local volunteers as community health workers and these also provide a valuable resource for health education.

What method will you use for reaching the intended audience?

A further set of choices concerns the educational methods to be used. Earlier decisions on target audiences and channels may have already determined the choice. For example if you choose to work through schools to reach young people your methods will probably involve classroom activities, educational projects and field visits. Some of the many different communication methods are shown in Figure 1.11.

Chapter 3 will review some of the advantages and disadvantages of different educational methods and the influence of source, method, channel and receiver on the effectiveness of communication.

What is the best timing for your programme?

You will have to decide on the best timing for your health promotion intervention. An intensive approach for a short time period is called a *campaign*. In a campaign it is often possible to involve large number of different groups for a short period of intensive activity. For example campaigns have been used for immunisation programmes in Latin America. In Honduras, a campaign using radio and leaflets to promote

Health services
doctors and nurses in primary
   health care
midwives
health visitors
public health nurses
village health workers
nutrition programmes
immunization programmes

Informal processes in the community
elders
parents and child-rearing
peers
traditional birth attendants
traditional healers
village leaders
religious leaders
non-governmental organisations

Public health services
public health inspectors
water supply
sanitation
hygiene inspection
refuse collection

Education services
teachers in primary and secondary
   schools
adult education
literacy programmes
pre-school programmes
vocational training

Agriculture and socio-economic development
agricultural extension
community development
applied nutrition programmes
cooperatives
employment-generating programmes
women's programmes

Fig. 1.10   Many people can be mobilised for improving the health of the
community

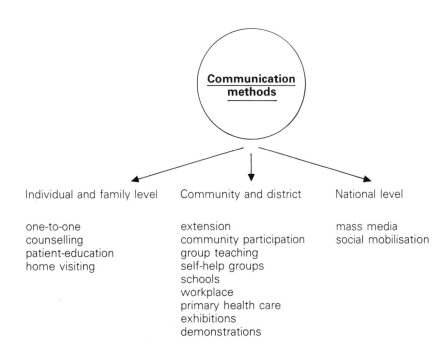

Fig. 1.11   Communication methods and health

oral rehydration was held at the start of the rainy season just before the peak period of diarrhoea. Another focus for campaigns is an 'international day' agreed by the United Nations – such as World AIDS Day on 1st December each year.

Some people are critical of the campaign approach because they feel that it is short-lasting. They claim that it is better to develop an 'on-going' programme that is 'institutionalised' into the daily work of services such as clinics, community health services and schools. Others find campaigns useful as a way of generating enthusiasm and involving a wide range of organisations in supporting their work.

Summary

You can see that actions to improve a community's health usually involve a combination of health education, service improvement and advocacy (HESIAD). Effective communication is a vital part of all three of these sets of activities.

Table 1.2 summarises some of these key decisions on approaches described above. Making these decisions will involve adopting a *systematic approach* to planning communication activities, which is set out in Figure 1.12. This will involve analysing the situation, studying the problem, gathering information on your communities and working out answers to the following questions.

- WHAT is the problem?
- WHAT are the causes of the problem?
- WHAT is the role of human behaviour?
- WHAT is the role of health education, service improvement and advocacy in dealing with the problem?
- WHO should the communication be directed at – i.e. the target group?

Table 1.2 Key areas of decision-making in communication and health education

Broad approach	Horizontal or vertical programme	Target groups	Level of operation	Channel or method for reaching target group/strategy	Time scale for activities undertaken
PERSUASIVE agency-determined objectives specific behavioural outcomes or HEALTH EMPOWERMENT educational empowerment decision-making participation	HORIZONTAL general lifestyle improvement or VERTICAL nutrition AIDS STDs alcohol tobacco drugs malaria schistosomiasis diarrhoea cancer family planning dental disease immunisation etc	women children men pregnant women parents of pre-school children elderly teenagers schoolchildren out-of-school youth college students health workers factory workers politicians opinion leaders etc.	individual family community district region national international	health services primary health care services schools mass media churches voluntary sector community project workplace intersectoral collaboration politicians self-help groups	SHORT-TERM intensive activity (campaign approach) LONGER TERM approach with greater integration

- WHAT approach to use:
  - persuasion or health empowerment?
  - single issue or broad-based health?
  - intensive campaign or ongoing programme?
- WHAT level (individual, family, community, national, international) should be used for the communication?
- WHAT setting/channel should be used to reach the intended audience?
- WHAT methods should be used?

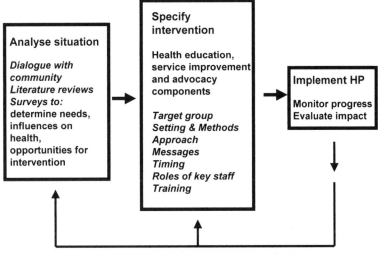

Fig. 1.12   Planning process for health promotion

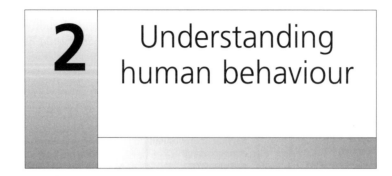

2 Understanding human behaviour

In Chapter 1 you saw how an important justification for health education and health promotion comes from the fact that health is determined, not by medical services and drugs, but by ordinary human actions and behaviours. Many health education programmes have failed because they neglected to understand the cultural, social, economic and political factors that influence these actions. Some people are critical of studying human behaviour and claim that this puts too much emphasis on individual action rather than the need for political, social and economic change. However, a proper understanding of the influences on human behaviour will avoid the pitfalls of victim blaming. It can do this by separating out those influences that are under the control of individuals from those that require actions at community and national level. Furthermore, fighting poverty, challenging injustice and working for political change are all 'behaviours' themselves. We need to understand the motivations that influence politicians to adopt policies and individuals to come together for community action and social change.

This chapter will therefore look at the following questions:

- What are behaviours and how can we describe them?
- What influences human behaviour?
- What is the role of culture, social change and economic factors in determining behaviours?

- How do we use an understanding of behaviour to plan health education and health promotion programmes?

Empathy – understanding other people's perspectives

We often complain because the community ignores our advice to follow healthy behaviours. Precautions to maintain health that make sense to us, are rejected by the community.

One reason for this is that we look at actions from our own point of view and place too much emphasis on health and medical factors as a reason for action. The community may consider other values to be more important, such as economic survival, status, prestige, physical beauty, attractiveness to the opposite sex, conforming to moral or religious rules and family honour. Our own motives, values, understandings may be very different from that of the community, especially if we come from different backgrounds. *What may seem to us as irrational behaviour by the community can actually involve deliberate and rational decisions based on the community's own perceptions of their situation and needs.*

The approach I use in this book assumes that people are not irrational or irresponsible but try to do what they see to be the best for themselves and their families. A useful approach is 'value expectancy theory' which suggests that people will only perform a given behaviour if *they themselves* see that it will provide some benefits, e.g. if they see that breastfeeding brings about mostly good outcomes they will wish to breastfeed. If they see breastfeeding brings about mostly bad outcomes they will not wish to breastfeed.

It is *the person's own judgement* of what is a good or bad outcome that matters. What is important to us may not be considered a worthwhile outcome by the community. What is important to the community may not be important to us – but we must still respect it. It is our task as health educators to ensure that the community's judgement is based on a sound understanding of the consequences of alternative actions.

A good example of the importance of understanding the community's perspective comes from the experiences in family planning programmes such as in India. Planners and health educators put effort into family planning because they were worried that the growing population was using up available resources. In their educational messages they emphasised national priorities and the cost of food, clothing and school fees. These issues were important to the planners and health educators who usually came from urban middle-class backgrounds.

However, as shown in Figure 2.1, the community viewed it differently. For poor people, having more children made good sense: extra children were more hands to help in the home and fields as well as sources of care and support in their old age. They also knew from experience that some of their children would probably die of childhood diseases so they needed to have extra children to make certain enough survived. As a result of evaluating these early experiences, many in India now feel that family planning programmes will only succeed if they are part of a general health programme and accompanied by measures attacking poverty.

To understand why people do or do not perform a particular behaviour we have to try to find out how the community – e.g. the pregnant woman, child, elderly person, village elder – *themselves* look at the action.

Imagine you are a villager. Consider one of the behaviours mentioned in the previous chapter such as breastfeeding, building a latrine, bringing a child for measles immunisation and coming for antenatal care. Write down what you think might appear to the villager as the benefits of performing the behaviour and compare them with what they might see as disadvantages. Now imagine you are a health worker

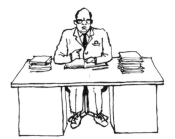

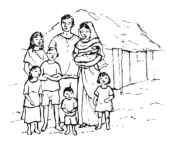

Planner's

If you have fewer children you will be able to spend more money on each and have a higher standard of living

You will have fewer mouths to feed

The country cannot produce enough food for everyone, build sufficient schools, provide health services and jobs

Individual's

More children will mean more help in the home and fields

We can send some to the city to work

Enough will survive to look after me in my old age

Fig. 2.1   Different perspectives on family planning

trying to promote the behaviour in the community. Are there any differences between the health worker and the community in the way they see advantages and disadvantages?

This process of putting ourselves in the other person's position is called empathy. People who have lived in cities or who have gone for further education, can find it difficult to understand how rural people think and feel. Chapter 4 will give examples how it is possible to use exercises such as role-plays to help ourselves understand the difference between the community's feelings and values and our own.

Defining the behaviour

A starting point for understanding the factors that influence people's decisions about adopting a behaviour is to define the behaviour in as much detail as possible. This involves specifying not only *what* the behaviour is but *who* is to carry it out and *when*.

It is difficult to analyse vaguely stated behaviours such as 'sanitation' – but easier with more precise statements that specify the type of latrine and required building materials. Terms such as 'hygiene practices' and 'family planning' apply to *groups* of behaviours. Family planning can include vasectomy, female sterilisation, condoms and the contraceptive pill. Hygiene includes washing of hands with soap, food preparation, clean storage of drinking water, disposal of infants' faeces. Each of these behaviours is influenced by different factors.

By specifying behaviours in detail, we can begin to consider some of the difficulties families face in putting our advice into practice. It is not enough just to say growth monitoring, immunisation, weaning and child spacing. By defining immunisation and growth monitoring in terms of a person bringing the child to a clinic it becomes obvious that you need to find out how accessible these services are and if mothers/caretakers have the time to bring the child. For weaning it is important to be clear what foods should be given, how frequently and when, and the need for continuing breast-feeding for as long as possible.

A good example of the importance of specifying the behaviour at the beginning of a programme is the use of oral rehydration solution (ORS) for children with diarrhoea. You will have to decide whether it is appropriate in that particular community to promote the use of packets or home-made solution. If home-made, you will have to decide whether to base it on salt/sugar, rice/other cereal solutions or readily available home fluids. You will also have to consider the type of containers to make up the solution, how much ORS to give and when to start giving it to the child. The World Health Organization now recommends that diarrhoea should be first treated in the home with any available fluid including water (some local 'bush' teas may not be suitable). ORS should only be used if there are signs of dehydration. Only when you have made these decisions on the type of ORS can you begin to analyse possible obstacles to adoption of ORS in your community and decide what you need to include in your educational programme.

You can begin to make judgements about the feasibility of changing a behaviour once you have described it carefully and considered the following questions:

A check-list for describing a behaviour
• How often should it be performed – daily, every few days, occasionally, only once?
• How complicated is it to carry out – is it very simple or does it require learning new skills?
• How similar is it to existing practices – is it completely new, or does it show some similarities?
• How easily does it fit in with existing practices – is it totally incompatible, partly compatible or does it fit in with existing practices?
• How much does it cost, in time, money or resources to carry out the behaviour?
• Does the behaviour fit in with a felt need of the community?
• How much impact will the behaviour have on health – a great deal, very little?
• Will beneficial effects be observed in the short or long term – within a few weeks, months or years?

You can predict a great deal from the answers to these questions. Hygiene behaviours such as cleaning children and washing hands have to be done every day. They will be more difficult to promote than a behaviour such as immunisation that only has to be done a few times. Behaviours which involve spending time or money, require learning new skills or conflict with existing practices will be more difficult to promote than ones that are simple to carry out and fit in with existing practices. *Customs* and *traditions* are behaviours that have been carried out for a long time and have been handed down from parents to children. They will be more difficult to change than behaviours that have been recently acquired and held only by individuals.

Sometimes our analysis of the influences on a behaviour will tell us that it is not realistic to attempt to promote a particular behaviour because of the enabling factors that would be required. A good example of this is boiling of drinking water. Boiling of drinking water requires a person's time for supervision and for the water to cool. Fuel is required which must be paid for or collected. A family must have a suitable cooking pot and an appropriate storage container for the water.

You will have more impact if you advise behaviours appropriate to people's income and culture. For example if people do not eat particular foods, you can develop nutrition advice that does not involve those foods. As a general rule you should make *your* advice fit the community rather than expect them to change to suit you.

Behavioural intention and enabling factors

You should try to avoid putting the blame for a failure of a health education programme on lack of interest or motivation on the part of the community. The distinguished health educator Lawrence Green developed a useful concept that he called *enabling factors*. Sometimes a person may intend to perform a behaviour but still not do so. This is because of the influence of enabling factors such as time, money, equipment, skills or health services.

Enabling factors for a mother to give oral rehydration solution to her child with diarrhoea would be: time, containers, salt and sugar and knowledge of how to prepare and administer it. Enabling factors for a latrine programme would be: money, essential components, e.g. slabs and the necessary construction skills. For a family planning programme enabling factors would be availability of contraceptives, accessible family

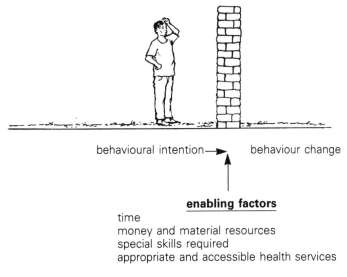

behavioural intention——→   behaviour change

enabling factors

time
money and material resources
special skills required
appropriate and accessible health services

Fig. 2.2   Enabling factors

planning services and the necessary skills on using the particular method. Convenient and accessible services are important enabling factors for the utilisation of child health services or antenatal clinics.

You should ensure that when the public makes the effort to follow your health education advice that the required services such as screening facilities, medicines, vaccines, building materials etc. are actually available.

Money can be another important enabling factor! Many health education programmes have failed because they did not consider the poverty and social inequalities that often underlie a particular behaviour. Social inequalities present a serious challenge to the improvement of health.

A neglected enabling factor is the *time* to carry out the health-promoting actions. Most of the important child care practices promoted in the 'Facts for Life' programme described in the previous chapter will require additional time caring for the child, taking to clinics, giving ORS etc. In most situations it is the mother who is expected to undertake these extra tasks. However, women in developing (and developed) countries are already overworked with *multiple roles* that include looking after the home, fetching water and fuel, caring for children, taking children to the child health clinic, preparing meals, growing food and going out to work. Their workload increases in particular seasons such as planting and harvesting when there is more agricultural work. These busy times of the year often coincide with seasonal peaks in food shortages and diseases such as diarrhoea. It is unrealistic to expect women to take action to improve health and nutrition unless we find ways of reducing their workload to give them time to follow our advice.

Social pressure

One reason health education programmes fail is that they are directed at individuals and ignore the influences of other people. Few people make decisions or perform actions without considering the opinions and views of

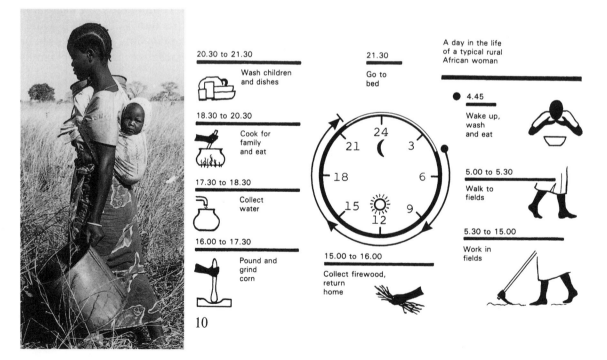

Fig. 2.3   A woman's work is never done

those around them. Think about your own family and friends. Whom do you consult when you have to make an important decision? As you can see in Figure 2.4, we are all influenced by the various persons in our *social network*. Some people may want you to take action – others may oppose you. Exactly who has the most influence will depend both on the particular individual and the culture of the community. For example, in some societies the mother-in-law is particularly influential; in others it may be the elders, including uncles.

The influential people – called *significant others* – change during a person's life. In a young child it is usually the parents who have the most influence. As a child grows older, friends become important and a young person can feel a powerful pressure to conform to the 'peer group'. Examples of the importance of social pressure are: the woman who does not adopt family planning because her husband disapproves; the young man who starts smoking because his friends encourage him to do so; the mother who wants to give oral rehydration solution to the child but the grandmother objects; the child who cleans his teeth because his mother insists; and the family who built a latrine because the religious leader in the community wanted them to do so.

Pressure from others can be a positive influence to adopt health-promoting practices as well as an obstacle. In real life we are constantly under pressure to act in different ways. Some people may approve of us doing something, others may be against. How we respond will depend on whose opinions have the most influence on us. For example a woman may believe that her friends and the health worker wish her to build a latrine but her father and husband do not want her to build a latrine. She is likely to conform to wishes of those most important to her. The term 'subjective norm' was introduced by the psychologist Fishbein to describe the overall perceived social pressure.

I have listed some questions that you can ask to find out the influences of social pressure in your community (see page 31).

Social learning theory

Many of the current ideas about influences on human decision-making have been influenced by social cognitive theory – especially the Social Learning Theory developed by the American psychologist Albert Bandura. He disagreed with earlier 'behaviourist' ideas that

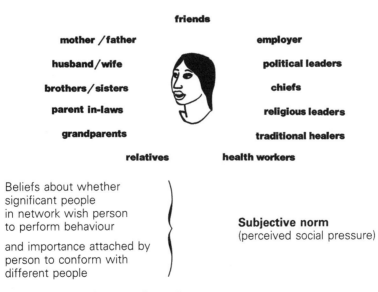

Fig. 2.4   The influence of social pressure

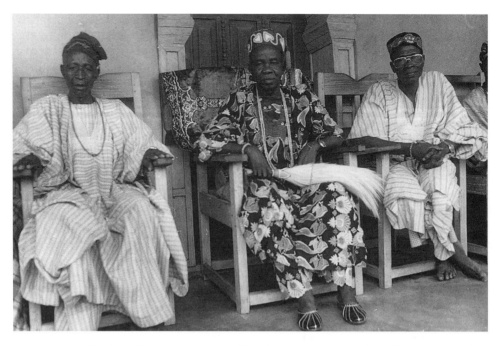

Fig. 2.5   An Oba (traditional chief) from Nigeria – an example of traditional authority

saw learning only as a result of external influences. Instead, he put forward the view that people learn not only through their own experiences, but also by observing the actions of others and the results of those actions. He suggested that each individual has a self-system and that human conduct is an interplay between the self-system and the environment. He considered that human activity had four special characteristics: the ability to symbolise their experiences, to learn from others, to regulate their own behaviour and to reflect on their own situation.

In this interaction between the individual and the environment he argues that it is people's beliefs about the world around them that have the most influence on their actions. Beliefs, according to Bandura, are: 'An individual's representation of reality that has enough personal validity and credibility to guide behavior and thought.' Beliefs affect human perception, interpretation and behaviour and therefore are the source of motivation. According to his theory an important influence on beliefs is through observing the actions of others – a process he called 'modelling'.

Of particular importance are the beliefs about oneself – the self concept. He went on to introduce the idea of self-efficacy : 'belief in one's capabilities to organize and execute the sources of action required to manage prospective situations.'

Social learning theory is important in health promotion because it emphasises the importance of understanding actions from the individual's perspective. The concept of self-efficacy is especially useful and is a key part of the health empowerment approach to promotion described in Chapter 1.

A related concept is that of self-esteem, which is the extent to which a person regards himself or herself to be of value. People with low self-esteem are considered easily persuaded by others, e.g. to perform harmful behaviours such as smoking, drinking and taking drugs. A person with high self-esteem is more able to resist pressures and able to do what they feel is right. Many people feel that the promotion of self-esteem is an important goal and this approach has been adopted widely especially in school health education and in work with disadvantaged groups.

Questions to ask to find out about social pressures	**Case studies of health promotion programmes based on an understanding of sources of influence**

Who are the most influential people in the community? Are there informal leaders who are looked to for decisions although they remain in the background? What qualities tend to make people's opinion carry weight in the community (money, children, age, education, cattle, wives)?

In what areas of life, e.g. economic, child care, food production, do the various leaders have influence? What leaders within the community are most likely to make decisions that influence community health, the delivery of health care in the area, or various aspects of the health programme? What do they think about the practices that you are trying to promote? Are there differences of views among the different leaders? Could local leaders be involved in your health education? How can you reach them?

How important is family membership in community life? How are families and kinship groups typically organised within the culture? What roles do the father, mother, son, daughter grandparents (or other persons typically part of the family within a certain culture) play within the family? Where and how does each member typically spend his time?

How and by whom are family decisions typically made? Who is consulted? What is the typical timing for various types of decisions? Where does the power within the family appear to lie? How do they feel about outsiders?

Who generally makes various health-related decisions within the family (i.e. what to do when a member is sick, whether to take certain preventive measures, what the family will eat, what money can be allotted for health-related expenses, whether a sick member may follow certain medical advice)?

Do children ever make health-related decisions? Are they taken seriously if their views differ from their parents?

Targeting husbands in family planning education in Ethiopia. Female health assistants accompanied by traditional birth attendants carried out two home visits to couples. The sessions started with a discussion on the health of the family and the woman's reproductive history. The content of the education focused on the advantages of family planning for preventing pregnancy, birth spacing and controlling family size. A follow-up survey found that impact of the education on uptake of contraception was higher when both partners were involved than when only the wife was given health education.

Involving Buddist monks' groups in anti-smoking education in Thailand. An anti-smoking campaign involved monks in a rural community to support the programme. An evaluation found that the proportion of smokers who were aware of the harmful effects of smoking and who had given up, was much greater in those communities compared with communities who did not have the programme.

Involving religious leaders in AIDS education in Uganda. The Islamic Medical Association of Uganda designed a 2-year AIDS prevention project and conducted a baseline survey before community level activities. Over 3000 religious leaders and their assistants were trained as 'Family AIDS Workers' who in turn educated their communities on AIDS during home visits and at religious gatherings. An evaluation showed an increase in knowledge, a reduction in self-reported sexual partners and a significant increase in self-reported condom use among males.

Culture and behaviour

Most people agree that culture has an important influence on behaviour. It is common to hear the terms cultural practice, cultural belief, cultural value and cultural norm. However, culture is a misunderstood term and actually consists of three overlapping features: shared characteristics, traditions and belief systems.

Shared characteristics

A behaviour, value or belief can be shared by a group of people, a whole community or even a country. The term sub-culture can also be applied to a group, such as teenagers, soldiers, factory workers, when we consider their special characteristics. Other words for shared characteristics are *norms or customs*, i.e. something that is common or normal for that group.

Traditions

These are practices that have been held for a long time and passed down from parents to children. Another word for this process of handing down from one generation to another is socialisation. 'Primary socialisation' is the term for the learning that takes place from one's family during the first 5 years. During this period the language, habits, values, beliefs and rules of behaviour of that society are learnt. This happens by the child following the instructions of the parent as well as the more informal process of copying the actions of adults.

Belief systems

While some behaviours exist on their own, others are part of wider system of beliefs such as

religion or a traditional medicine system. For example, in one person avoidance of pork may be simply a matter of not liking the taste. In another person that behaviour might be because the person is a Jew or Muslim.

We can apply these three components of culture – shared characteristics, traditions and a system of beliefs to the processes listed here which all influence health and health education activities.

Health – an ancient concept rooted in culture

Health itself is a concept determined by culture and society and we may each have our own ideas about what it means to be healthy. Health is so important to basic functions of survival that it is not very surprising that most societies in the world have well-established ideas about health.

In looking at these definitions of health some significant points emerge. Despite the broad nature of the WHO definition, many doctors and health workers still see health in terms of

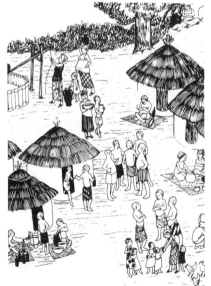

A great deal is learnt during early years from the family – this process is called primary socialisation.

Fig. 2.6 Traditions and norms

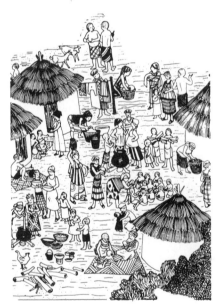

Many characteristics are shared by different people in a community – norms.

Different ways in which culture can influence health	**Some definitions of health**

Different ways in which culture can influence health

- **Life cycle**: family structure, patterns of influence among family members, role of women, children, rituals and roles surrounding birth, growing up, relations with other people, sex and marriage; family formation, work, growing old, death.
- **Patterns of living and consumption**: clothing; housing; child rearing, food production, storage and consumption; hygiene practices; sanitation.
- **Health and illness behaviours**: concepts of health and illness; ideas about mental illness and handicap; care of sick people; traditional medicine systems; patterns of help-seeking when ill; use of doctors and traditional healers; concepts about the biological workings of the body, growth, conception, pregnancy, birth etc.
- **Patterns of communication**: language; verbal and non-verbal communication; taboos on public discussion of sensitive items; vocabulary of the language; oral traditions.
- **Religion and 'world view'**: ideas about the meaning of life and death; rituals surrounding important life events; ideas about the possibility and desirability of change.
- **Patterns of social and political organisation**: political structures; community leadership and authority; divisions and social inequalities.
- **Economic patterns types of employment**: ideas about wealth and income; ownership of land; use of money and barter; savings and credit arrangements.

Some definitions of health

'A state of complete physical, mental and social well-being, not merely the absence of disease or infirmity.' WHO (1946)

'The nearest approach to health is a physical and mental state fairly free of discomfort and pain, which permits the person concerned to function as effectively and as long as possible in the environment where chance or choice has placed him.' Dubos

'The Yoruba generic concept for health is *Alafia*. In its literal sense *Alafia* means peace. The word embraces the totality of an individual's physical, social, emotional, psychological and spiritual well-being in the total environmental setting. The Yorubas believe that the possession of *Alafia* is a result of the dynamic interaction of all those variables. According to the people: "*Eni ba l'Alafia l'ohun gbogbo*" (Whoever has health has all things) and "*Alafia l'ogun oso*" (Health is wealth).' Ademuwagun (1978) Nigeria

'According to Indian philosophy, the universe consists of five gross elements – earth, water, fire, air and the ethereal parts of the sky – and the same factors constitute the basic elements of the human body. However, in a human body, life does not depend only on these five bodily components but also on the presence of normally functioning sense organs and of the mind and soul. Thus Sushruta refined the healthy person as follows: "He is the healthy man who possesses the balance of body hormones, proper functioning of all the body elements and who has the pleasant disposition of mind, soul and sense organs."' Valupa (1975)

diseases and disease prevention. However, traditional ideas of health in Asian, African and European cultures have a wider *holistic* view. Health can be:

- a feeling of well-being;
- opportunity of achieving fulfilling activities;
- a balance of physical and mental states;
- achievement of one's potential; or
- ability to cope with life's demands.

Many different traditional medicine systems are practised throughout the world.

Traditional healers may be widely respected and are consulted by a wide range of people. In the past they were criticised and called quacks and witch doctors. It is now realised that they have an important role to play and that efforts should be directed towards integrating them within primary health care. Some of the questions you will need to find out in your community about health systems are listed here.

Concepts of health and illness – a checklist of questions

Concepts of health and illness: What factors do people in the community generally consider make up a state of wellness/good health or illness/poor health? What conditions of the body are considered normal and abnormal? What is considered to be a physical 'handicap'? What are their feelings towards people who have abnormalities or are disabled? What priority does the value of 'good health' have within the community? How important is health compared with other needs and values?

Coping with illness: What types of actions do families take when a member becomes ill or injured? Are particular family or community members involved in the prevention, diagnosis or treatment of certain illnesses of other family members? Are there special family medicines, remedies, treatments? Do family health beliefs and practices differ from your health education messages?

What are the typical attitudes within a culture toward the sick? Who decides within a culture if a person is ill? How is the sick person expected to behave? Does the person consult family or traditional healers first before consulting western practitioners? What methods do traditional healers use?

Beliefs about health, disease, treatment and prevention: What general beliefs do various community people have concerning cause, prevention, diagnosis and treatment of diseases in general or specific ones? Are there any particular methods people use to help maintain their own health or that of others? Are there any special traditional theories of disease to which certain people adhere? Do they still believe them? What is the general understanding of and attitude towards Western medical explanations and practices?

What are the attitudes of persons of various ages, sexes, ethnic groups and religions towards the body? Towards discussing the body? Towards self-examination? What beliefs do people have concerning the organs and systems of the body and how they function?

General beliefs concerning health and illness behaviours: What are people's beliefs concerning immunisations, various screening tests, preventive health measures, hygiene, prevention of accidents and other behaviours you may be trying to promote in the community?

Are there any special beliefs, rules, preferences or prejudices concerning foods? Are foods used to treat diseases? What do the people feel should be an ideal diet? Does this change at different ages and special states, e.g. pregnancy?

How is knowledge concerning sex acquired by growing children? What are the social and cultural beliefs and practices surrounding sexual intercourse (premarital intercourse, contacting sex partners, homosexuality, bisexuality, techniques of sexual intercourse, sexual restrictions and extramarital intercourse)?

There are many different kinds of traditional medicine. Some of these, including the Hindu Ayurvedic medicine, the Chinese Yin/Yang system and homeopathic medicine are complex medical 'systems' with written books, training colleges and registration procedures for recognition. Others are small scale, informal and passed on through oral traditions and healers taking on 'apprentices' to study under them. The anthropologist George Foster suggests that traditional medical systems can be grouped into the two categories in Table 2.1. The first group, 'personalistic', includes systems of medicine where the blame for illness is put on supernatural forces, witchcraft, spirits or the 'evil eye'. In the second group, 'naturalistic', reasons for illness are based on 'natural' explanations including theories of the body, actions of herbs etc.

Values

Values are characteristics held to be important and prized by an individual or community. Usually values are qualities at an abstract level such as bravery and intelligence. A person's values might be reflected in the way he or she completes the following statement: *the things that are important to me are...* Examples of characteristics that can be valued by communities include:

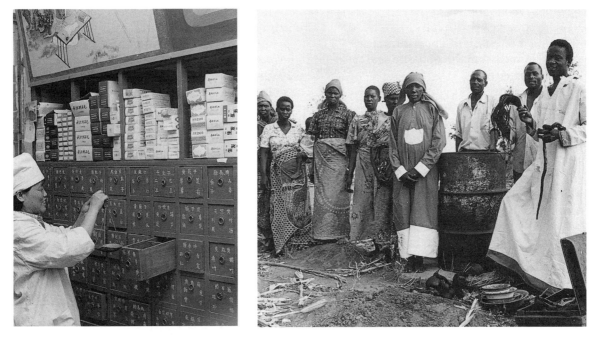

Fig. 2.7   Traditional healers: China (left) and Zambia (right)

Table 2.1   Types of traditional medical systems

	Supernatural	'Natural' explanations
Illness explained by	Active purposeful intervention of another person or supernatural agent, e.g. through witchcraft, evil eye, spirits	Explanations not based on supernatural influences but in terms of concepts of health and disease, e.g. lack of balance of factors in body, hot/cold theories, yin/yang etc.
Extent to which same explanation for illness also applies for other misfortunes	Illness is only a special case of a wider misfortune	Explanations limited to disease only, not other disasters or misfortunes
Levels of causation	Thinking about causes on different levels – not just cause of illness but who has caused it	Single level of cause – do not ask questions such as: Who caused the disease?
Diagnosis	Powerful witch doctors or spiritualists needed to identify who had caused the illness. Treatment less important	Patient seeks aid from curers for relief of symptoms and not to find out what has happened
Nature of curers	Curers are needed who have supernatural or magical divining power	Curers tend to be 'doctors' in that they have learnt their skills through observation and practice and not through divine intervention

- being a good mother
- being approved by friends
- having the respect of my community
- being attractive to the opposite sex
- being 'modern'
- being healthy
- having many children
- owning a large number of cattle
- being strong
- masculinity and sexual prowess

A person may have his or her own individual values. However, values are usually part of culture and shared at a community or national level. Health is only one of many possible values and a person may feel that other values such as fame, wealth or respect in the community may be more important.

We can sometimes bring about changes by emphasising values that do not involve health. For example we might explain to a woman that breastfeeding her child will bring her weight down after delivery and make her look more attractive. We might persuade a person to build a latrine by emphasising the benefits of privacy or of being considered modern by one's neighbours.

In health education we are often trying to promote health as a value or to encourage people to think about their values. This process is called *value-clarification* and is usually carried out through small group discussion.

It is important to avoid imposing your own values on the community – base your messages on what people *themselves* feel to be important.

Beliefs

Beliefs deal with a people's understanding of themselves and their environment. Beliefs about the different possible outcomes from performing actions are especially important in understanding behaviour. I list some types of beliefs that are important in health education as well as examples of each.

How beliefs are formed

It is important to find out how a particular belief has been acquired in order to predict how easy it might be changed. A belief might have been formed from an individual or community's personal experiences, e.g. they may have visited a

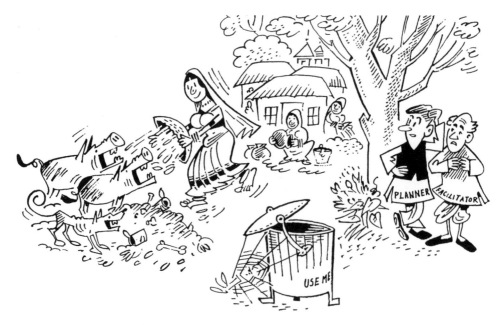

Fig. 2.8 Planners and facilitators must strive to understand the beliefs that influence behaviour... (SEARO cartoon)

Types of beliefs important in promotion of health	
Causes of diseases	*Lung cancer is caused by smoking.* *Accidents are caused by sorcery.*
How easily prevented a disease is	*Using a pit latrine will prevent hookworm.* *Immunisation will prevent measles.* *Methods for prevention of having children do not exist.*
Effort involved in taking action	*Building a pit latrine costs a lot of money.* *The health centre is very far away.*
Benefits resulting from taking action	*Taking part in a primary health care programme will improve our village.*
Consequences of disease	*Measles does not lead to death.* *Diarrhoea causes death.*
Personal susceptibility to 'disease'	*My children will not catch measles.* *I am not likely to get pregnant again.*
What is normal or a state of disease	*Malaria is very common here.* *Most people have six children.* *Diarrhoea is a normal state of growing up.*
What other persons think you should do	*My husband would disapprove of my using family planning.*
Beliefs about the possibility of change	*There is nothing I can do to grow more food.* *Having children is the will of God and I cannot change it.*
Credibility of communication source	*The nurse does not care about my baby.* *Our village level worker knows very little.*
Beliefs about prestige/status	*Bottle-feeding is practised by modern women.* *Building a pit latrine will make people look up to me.*

latrine and found it smelly; tried a folk remedy and felt better afterwards; attended a clinic and found long queues; seen a child receive an immunisation and then get measles (e.g. through poorly-kept vaccines), etc. It is difficult to change those beliefs that have arisen through a person's direct experience unless you can provide a practical demonstration.

The study of medical anthropology provides valuable insights into how particular beliefs can be part of wider belief systems such as religions and traditional medical systems. If a belief is part of a wider system of beliefs it can be very difficult to change, e.g. a pregnant woman in the Indian sub-continent might hold the belief that she should not eat eggs as part of a general concept of hot/cold states of the body and foods.

A person also develops beliefs from what he/she reads or hears from other persons. For example, many beliefs are acquired during childhood from our parents and others in our family or community through *primary socialisation*. At each stage of the human life cycle from pre-school, school, to young adult upwards beliefs can be formed. It can be difficult to change those beliefs that have been held for a long time since childhood or have been acquired from trusted persons in the community.

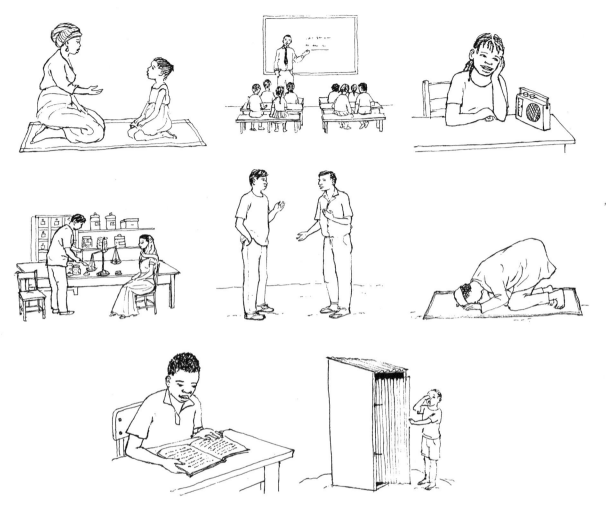

Fig. 2.9   Our beliefs have many origins – which do you think might be more difficult to change?

The Health Belief Model

The Health Belief Model (HBM) was developed by Rosenstock and Becker to explain why people did not use health services (utilisation behaviour), but has been applied to many aspects of health behaviour as well. According to the HBM, if a person is to perform a particular act such as going for cancer screening, he/she has to:

believe they are *susceptible*	that the health problem could affect him or her personally – rather than other people or society as a whole.
feel that it was *serious*	that the health problem, disease could lead to death or other serious outcomes if action was not taken.
believe it could be *prevented*	that taking the action would prevent the health problem and that the benefits of taking action would outweigh the disadvantages.

A man may accept alcoholism as serious and that it can be prevented but may not believe that *he* was susceptible and could become an alcoholic. Then you should not waste effort emphasising the seriousness of alcoholism but concentrate on making him realise that he could be at risk. A woman may believe that her child could get measles and that this would have serious consequences. However, she may not believe that measles can be prevented by immunisation. In that case you should base your communications strategy on promoting the belief that immunisation prevents measles.

The Health Belief Model provides a useful checklist for choosing the points to emphasise in any communication message – especially the importance of perceived seriousness, susceptibility and preventability. But it has some weaknesses: it does not consider social pressure from others in the family or community and ignores enabling factors. These are both taken into account in the BASNEF Model described in the next section.

Attitudes and Fishbein

Attitudes and beliefs are frequently confused. The psychologist Martin Fishbein suggested that the term attitude should be used for a person's judgement of a behaviour as good or bad and worth carrying out. This judgement will depend on the beliefs held about the consequences of performing the behaviour. A person will normally hold a range of beliefs about the possible good and bad consequences of performing a particular behaviour. For example a mother may believe that breastfeeding will improve the health of her baby but may also believe that it will make her appear old-fashioned. If, overall, a person believes that performing the behaviour will lead to mainly good outcomes, then the attitude will be favourable. If the outcomes are perceived as mainly bad, the attitude to the behaviour will be unfavourable.

Whether the overall judgement (i.e. attitude) of the behaviour is favourable or unfavourable will also depend on the values placed on the different possible consequences, e.g. in the latrine example the values placed on health, privacy, owning a bicycle, foul smells, flies, appearing

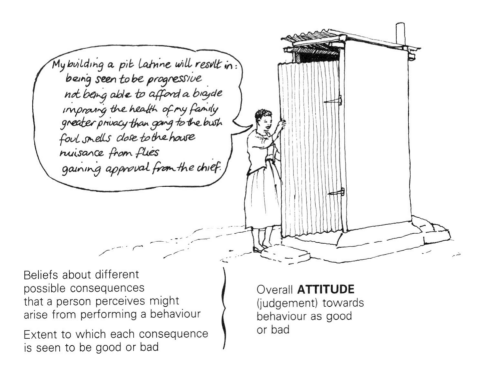

Beliefs about different possible consequences that a person perceives might arise from performing a behaviour

Extent to which each consequence is seen to be good or bad

Overall **ATTITUDE** (judgement) towards behaviour as good or bad

Fig. 2.10   Role of beliefs in forming attitude

progressive etc. A particular consequence may be perceived as a bad one by one person, but acceptable (and even an advantage!) by another person.

According to Fishbein, whether or not a person forms an intention to perform a behaviour will also depend on the overall pressure from those around him, i.e. *subjective norm*. A person may judge the proposed behaviour favourably but may perceive that those important to him do not want him to perform the behaviour. A person may not have a favourable attitude towards the behaviour but be pressurised by those around him to perform it.

Whether or not the person's own judgement can overcome the influence of those around him will depend on the individual's strength of will and susceptibility to pressure. There can be considerable cultural pressure on individuals to conform to family and community influence.

Fishbein incorporated his concept of attitude with that of subjective norm into a model of behaviour that he called the Theory of Reasoned Action. It was a significant improvement on the Health Belief Model because it considers both an individual's beliefs as well as the social pressures from others in the family and community.

Putting it all together – BASNEF

I have put together the BASNEF model (the name comes from the first letters of Beliefs, Attitude, Subjective Norm and Enabling Factor) by combining the approach by Fishbein discussed in the previous section and the concept of Enabling Factors introduced by Lawrence Green; it is summarised in Figure 2.11. It should be seen as a checklist for programme planning rather than a complete description of the complex processes that underlie a person's actions. An implication of this model is that people may react differently to a particular message depending on their beliefs, social pressures or the presence or absence of enabling factors (see Figure 2.12).

Stages of change theory

The Stages of Change Theory, also called the Transtheoretical Theory, was put forward by two Americans Prochaska and DiClemente and is now being applied in many situations. The basis of this theory is that behaviour change is a process that takes place over time. The theory shares some features of Communication of Innovations Theory which is described in

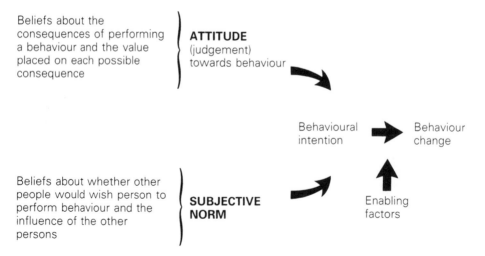

Fig. 2.11   Summary of BASNEF model for understanding behaviour

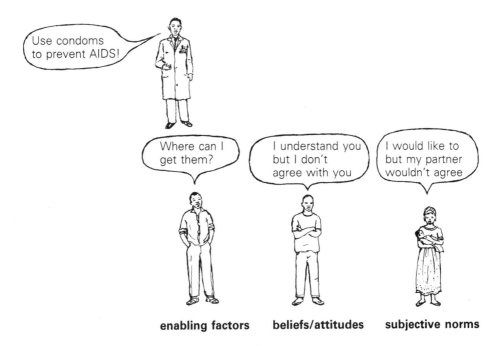

Fig. 2.12   Three possible reactions to a talk

Case studies of health promotion programmes that take into account local beliefs

Multimedia family planning campaign in Bamako, Mali to influence beliefs about family planning: An integrated multimedia campaign featuring family planning messages saturated the 900,000-person city of Bamako, Mali, for 3 months. Alongside traditional theatre and music, family planning messages were repeatedly broadcast on radio and television about modern contraceptive methods, the need for male sexual responsibility, the health and economic advantages of family planning and that Islam, the predominant faith of Mali, does not oppose family planning. The evaluation showed a large drop in the proportion of the community who believed that Islam opposes family planning and a greater stated willingness to use modern of contraceptives in future.

Involving traditional healers in Brazilian urban slums in prevention of AIDS in Northeast Brazil. During a 12-month period Afro-Brazilian Umbanda healers taught 126 fellow healers from seven slums about safe sex practices, avoidance of ritual blood behaviours, and sterilisation of cutting instruments. An evaluation found that, when compared with healers who had not received training, trained healers had significantly higher levels of awareness about AIDS, condom use and risky behaviours. They were also more prepared to accept lower-risk alternative ritual blood practices.

Community-based schistosomiasis control in North Province, Cameroon. A survey was used to find out existing understanding and words used for schistomiasis. The information collected was used to design an educational programme which involved religious and political leaders and also community groups including women's associations. Other activities included development of materials (flip chart, posters and brochures) training of primary school teachers and health workers. Overall prevalence of infection declined from 21% to 7%.

Community-based HIV/AIDS education in Moyo District, Uganda. A survey of knowledge, attitudes and practice was carried out and the information gathered used to design a programme and supporting materials, including a leaflet. Groups of 30 community educators were recruited from every parish in the district and trained to conduct information sessions at the village level. During the first 5 months of the information campaign an estimated 50,000 people attended the village-based information sessions and 45,000 pamphlets and 40,000 condoms were distributed. A survey found that knowledge about condoms and reported use had increased in the programme area.

Radio soap opera in St Lucia, West Indies.
A research programme identified 37 issues affecting family planning and sexual health which included knowledge, attitudes and behaviour related to family planning, HIV prevention, gender equity, relationship fidelity and domestic violence. These were incorporated into a radio drama series – more than 300 episodes of Apwe Plezi were broadcast over 3 years. The characters served as positive and negative role models and the story lines raised issues identified in the initial research and showed the consequences of the different behaviours of the characters. The radio drama was accompanied by other educational activities including street theatre performed 21 times, reports in the local newspaper, posters, bumper stickers and billboards. The radio drama launched a new name for condoms – 'catapult'. An evaluation confirmed the popularity of the programme, its impact on knowledge and attitudes and awareness of the new name for condoms.

Chapter 3. According to the Stages of Change Theory, in a given community people may be at different stages in the process of change – see below and also Figure 2.13.

- *Pre-contemplation* – The person has not thought about changing and may not be aware of risks of current behaviour. Not interested in changing behaviour.
- *Contemplation* – The person is aware of some of the benefits of changing and is thinking about changing.
- *Decision* – The person has made a decision to change and is ready to adopt new practice.
- *Action* – The person has made the change.
- *Maintenance* – The change has been included into the person's lifestyle as part of his or her regular routine behaviour.

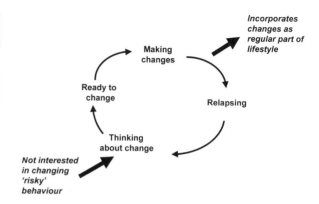

Fig. 2.13   The stages of change model

Many of the factors discussed earlier in this chapter, such as beliefs, enabling factors and social pressure, may apply at each of these stages. A useful part of the theory is that it is expressed as a cycle. A person may change their behaviour but later return to old practices. They may go round the cycle several times before finally incorporating the change into their lives.

The Stages of Change Theory has some practical implications. Different people may be at different stages. You need to find out at what stage a person is and tailor the health education message accordingly. Questions that could be asked to find out what stage a person is at could include:

Have you thought about ... . . (e.g. quitting smoking, using a latrine, using a condom)
Are you thinking about ... . . soon?
Are you ready to ... ... ?
Are you in the process of ... ... ?
Are you trying to continue ... ... ?
Did you try ... ... and give it up?

In a community there may be people at different stages and no single approach will be relevant for everyone. As well as targeting people who have not changed, the theory suggests that you need to also to target those who have already changed – to give them support and encouragement so that they do not return to their old practices.

Using an understanding of behaviour to promote health

Applying the approaches described above involves examining the behaviour from the perspective of the community. This is not as easy as it sounds as, even if you share their background, your education and health training will make you look at issues differently. You will need to speak to individuals and groups at the beginning of a health education session to find out about the underlying factors including beliefs, values, social pressure and enabling factors that influence the community. You can use the questions in the lists on social influence, health beliefs as well as the lists of beliefs to form the basis for choosing what questions to answer. If resources are available, you can carry out this questioning more systematically as an organised survey or 'community diagnosis'.

Once sufficient background information is available on the various factors influencing behaviour, making decisions on health education and health promotion approaches involves the steps below (see also Figure 2.14).

1. **Make sure the behaviour will improve health**. Before devoting time and energy to promoting a behaviour, make sure that it will actually benefit the community. It is still common to find health educators wasting effort trying to persuade people to give up harmless behaviours or take up new behaviours for which there is little evidence of health benefits.
2. **Make sure the behaviour change you are asking for is a realistic one.** Avoid behaviours that are complicated, require enabling factors such as time, money, new skills and do not fit in with the culture and present practices.

    Can the proposed behaviour be changed to make it more acceptable, cheaper and easier to carry out? You might be able to reduce the cost by developing low-cost solutions such as cheaper latrines, heat-efficient ovens etc. An *appropriate technology* should be compatible with the culture of the community, technically feasible using locally available skills and materials, require minimum maintenance and be simple to use. For example, in the case of sanitation, if your analysis of culture and beliefs indicates that the community prefer sitting to squatting, you should design latrines with seats. If it is acceptable to build latrines in a spiral shape without doors you can avoid the cost of doors.

3. **Provide necessary enabling factors**. Your intervention plan should make sure that the required enabling factors are available. This could involve setting up community organisation programmes aimed at improving living conditions such as income, housing, water supply, agriculture and sanitation. It may be necessary to improve the situation of women to provide the additional time required to carry out the behaviour. Services could be improved to make them accessible and more appropriate, e.g. more convenient times, outreach into communities, improved confidentiality and training of field staff to improve their rapport with communities. You can also include opportunities for the community to learn any special skills needed to put the advice into practice.

    By careful questioning, you can find out whether enabling factors are needed. A good example of this is the question that the nutritionist Judith Brown asks first when planning a nutrition intervention. *Does the family have sufficient resources to grow or buy the necessary food?*

    If NO Then tackle the food availability issue first and find ways of improving their economic position so that they can obtain the food.

    If YES Then explore other reasons why they may not prepare the food such as lack of time, necessary knowledge or beliefs.

Tackling enabling factors can involve moving well beyond the traditional range of activities for health services. This often involves *intersectoral collaboration* – working with field personnel from other services such as agriculture, rural development, adult education and cooperatives. You may have to challenge vested interests at the local level and become involved in advocacy at a national level to influence government policies.

4. **Consider social pressures from the family and community**. If the enabling factors are all readily available, then the barrier to change may be social pressure on the person – the subjective norm. It is unreasonable to expect a person, no matter how convinced, to go against the wishes of those around him or her in the community. Giving advice to the individual at the clinic would not be enough. You must go into the community and convince the influential 'opinion leaders' in the family and community. For example you could set up demonstration latrines at their homes. You could look for opinion leaders who have successfully changed their lifestyle and would be happy to talk to others and explain the benefits of giving up smoking, using oral rehydration therapy, using a latrine, adopting child spacing etc. People are more easily persuaded by people they trust and believe. These 'satisfied acceptors' can be a powerful help in your educational programmes.

5. **Identify any beliefs that might influence the person's attitude**. The blame for failure has often been put on 'bad beliefs' and 'laziness' and health education programmes often fail to take into account the enabling factors and social pressure described above.

   If the community believes that performing the behaviour will lead to unfavourable outcomes you should try to find out why. You might be able to change the proposed behaviour to make it more acceptable. If this is not possible – and there is clear evidence of health benefits from changing the behaviour – then it is justifiable to try to change beliefs. You could try to strengthen those beliefs that link performing the behaviour to outcomes that the community considers desirable.

   Earlier in this chapter I discussed the origins of beliefs and showed how you can predict which beliefs are the easiest to change. If it is just the individual who holds a particular belief then it might be possible to influence the belief by discussions only with

that person. More often, however, the belief is also held by others in the community as part of their shared culture. It is then necessary to direct effort at groups of people rather than individuals.

The community is more likely to be convinced if the benefits of a behaviour can clearly be shown in an observable demonstration, e.g. that a well-designed latrine does not smell, immunisation is effective, oral rehydration therapy prevents death. It is usually easier to influence those beliefs that have only been acquired recently, are held by individuals and not by the whole community, come from sources that are not highly respected and are not part of a religion or traditional medical system.

An important set of beliefs to target are those concerned with self-efficacy, which were discussed in the section on social learning theory. You will need to convince the community not only that change is important but also that they have the power to make those changes.

6. **Find out whether the influences on behaviour operate at the individual, family, community or higher level**. Health education can be criticised for over-emphasising working with individuals and failing to work at other levels such as the family, community, national and international level where many influences on behaviour operate (see Figure 1.8).

   Many of the problems of selection of unrealistic, inappropriate messages and behaviour changes can be resolved by working at the community level and building in community participation in the selection of objectives. Working at this level can create opportunities to for health empowerment. If it is necessary that traditional practices must change, then it is important that the community themselves make the decisions as to how these changes should take place.

7. **Advocacy.** Poor health may be because of problems at a community level or national decisions. Other influences at the national level are agricultural policies or commercial advertising. You may have to try to

influence governments to adopt health-promoting policies such as the restriction of health-damaging activities such as the advertising of baby milk and tobacco. The use of non-formal education techniques to generate community participation, raise consciousness and stimulate action on social and economic determinants of health will be described further in Chapter 6 'Working with communities' and Chapter 10 'Politics and health'.

Summary

This chapter has reviewed influences on human behaviour and has brought these together in an approach I have called BASNEF. The starting point for our analysis has been the individual person's behaviour. However, an understanding of the influences on behaviour can lead to interventions that go beyond the individual to include programmes at the family, community and national levels and involve health education, service improvement and advocacy for educational, social, economic and political change.

1 Have you drawn upon available current knowledge to make sure that the behaviours chosen will have an impact on prevention?
2 Can you choose behaviours that are:
   • simple to carry out and require few additional skills or resources?
   • compatible with local culture and acceptable to the community?
   • meet a felt need in the community and are wanted?
   • produce some benefits in the short term that are observable?
3 Are enabling factors such as money, time and materials required for performing the behaviour? If so, how can we make sure that they are provided through improving services, reducing costs?
4 If your programmes involve targeting women, have you taken into account the workload of women in the home and fields and other gender barriers?
5 Who are the significant persons in the family or community who have influence over the particular behaviour? Do they support your programme?
6 What beliefs does the community have about the consequences of performing the behaviour?

Influences

	Actions needed
culture / values / traditions / mass media / education / experiences **BELIEFS ATTITUDES**	Health education to modify beliefs and values of individuals or whole community
health services / income/poverty / inequalities / gender barriers / discrimination / employment / agriculture / transport **ENABLING FACTORS**	Service improvement to promote acceptability, effectiveness and quality: Advocacy to raise profile of issues, influence policy and promote intersectoral collaboration; skill training
family / community / social network / culture / social change / power structures / family structure **SUBJECTIVE NORM** (social pressure)	Health education targeted at influential persons in family and community

Fig 2.14 Influences on behaviour and choice of communication strategies

How were these beliefs formed? Can the unfavourable perceptions be reduced? Can the positive beliefs be strengthened?

7   Should you direct your efforts at the individual, family, district, national or international level?

8   How can you encourage community participation in the understanding of behaviour and planning of health education programmes?

9   What changes in government policy are needed to make healthy choices easier?

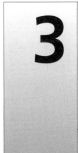

3 An introduction to communication

Communication involves the transfer between people of information including ideas, emotions, knowledge and skills. This chapter will:

1 Explore the psychological and social processes involved in communication, reasons for communication failure and provide guidelines for successful communication.
2 Examine the relative influences of source, message, channel and receiver on the communication process and consider how this understanding can help in designing communication programmes.
3 Consider how an understanding of pictures and visual perception can help in designing visual communications and audio-visual aids.
4 Explore the main characteristics of a range of communication methods – in particular face-to-face and mass media.
5 Provide a theoretical basis for later chapters in this book that look at the role of communication in teaching, mass media, community participation, working with people and use of folk media.

Communication stages

Communication can involve ordinary conversation, such as explaining a point, asking a question or just talking to pass the time. However, in health education and health promotion we communicate for a special purpose – to promote improvements in health through the modification of the human, social and political factors that influence behaviours and promote informed decision-making. To achieve these objectives, a successful communication must pass through several stages (Figure 3.2) – and at each stage communication failure can take place (see Table 3.1).

Stage 1: reaching the intended audience

Communication cannot be effective unless it is seen or heard by its intended audience. This may seem obvious and does not require any complex theories to explain. But many programmes fail even at this simple stage. A common cause of failure is *preaching to the converted*, e.g. posters placed at the clinic or talks given at the antenatal clinics. These only reach the people who attend the services and are already motivated.

But the groups you are trying to reach may not attend clinics, have radios or newspapers. They may be busy working at the time when the health education programmes are broadcast. Communications should be directed where people are going to see them or hear them. This requires studying your intended audience to find out where they might see posters, what their listening and reading habits are.

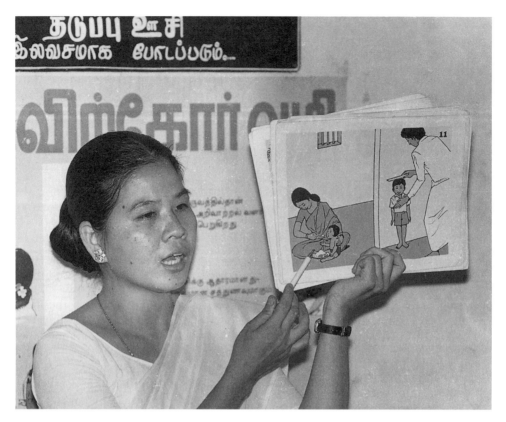

Fig. 3.1   Human communication

Stage 2: attracting the audience's attention

Any communication must attract attention so that people will make the effort to listen/read it. Examples of communication failures at this stage are:

- walking past the poster without bothering to look at it;
- not paying attention to the health talk or demonstration at the clinic;
- not stopping at the exhibition at the show-ground; and
- turning off the radio programme or switching over.

At any one time we receive a wide range of information from each of our five senses – touch, smell, sight, hearing and taste. It is impossible to concentrate on all this at the same time. Attention is the name of the process by

which a person selects part of this complex mixture to focus on (i.e. *to pay attention to*) while ignoring others for the time being. Some of the psychological processes that influence the way a

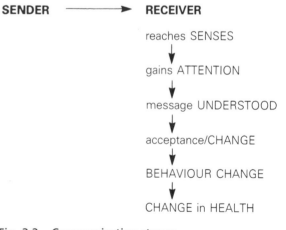

Fig. 3.2   Communication stages

Table 3.1 Examples of failure at different communication stages

	Immunisation poster	Water/ sanitation	Radio nutrition	How to ensure success
Reaches SENSES; is seen or heard	Poster is placed at the health centre and only seen by mothers who have already immunised their children	Only men, not women, were at the public meeting. The women did not hear about water programme	The radio programme was broadcast at a time when the women were working in the fields	*Research target group to find out where they go, what are their listening, viewing, reading habits*
Gains ATTENTION; holds interest, is noticed	The poster lacks striking features and does not stand out compared with attractive commercial advertisements	The sanitation exhibition at the agricultural show was boring so most people walked past	The nutrition programme was boring, so the women switched to the other station	*Find out interests of target group. Make programme interesting, attractive, and unusual. Test it out*
Is UNDERSTOOD; correctly interpreted	Poster showing large hypodermic syringe held by smiling doctor was thought by the community to be a devil with a knife	The fieldworker used complicated words such as faecal-borne diseases, stools and bacteria. No one understood	The women were confused by the technical terms, vitamins, proteins and xerophthalmia	*Make it simple, avoid confusing language. Pre-test words and pictures with sample of intended target group*
Is ACCEPTED, believed; learning takes place	People believe that measles is caused by witchcraft and do not believe the poster even though they understand the message	The fieldworker explained that diseases were passed by bacteria and faeces. The people laughed at this explanation	The announcer was a young girl and the women did not believe that she could know anything about children	*Base message on what people already believe. Use credible sources. Pre-test messages for acceptability*
CHANGES BEHAVIOUR	The mother accepted the message and wished to take child for immunisation but the grandmother did not allow it	They were convinced of the importance of pit latrines and wanted to build them. But they did not have any cement for slabs	The women wanted to put the advice into practice but did not have money to buy the food	*Target the influential people and ensure enabling factors are available. Pre-test for feasibility*
IMPROVES HEALTH	The vaccine was destroyed by a break in the cold chain and the child became sick with measles	They followed the advice and built latrines. But the children were afraid to use them so the levels of diarrhoea did not reduce	The women followed the advice and bought their children expensive protein foods – but stopped breastfeeding. The children developed malnutrition	*Choose most important behaviours. Make sure support services are functioning*

message can attract an audience's attention will be discussed later in this chapter.

Stage 3: understanding the message (perception)

Once a person pays attention to a message he/she then tries to understand it. Another name for this stage is perception. *Visual perception* is the term used for understanding of visual messages and *pictorial perception* for understanding of pictures. Perception is a highly *subjective* process – two people may hear the same radio programme or see the same poster or and interpret the message quite differently from each other and from the meaning intended by the sender.

A person's interpretation of a communication will depend on many things. Misunderstandings can easily take place when: complex language and unfamiliar technical words are used; pictures contain complicated diagrams, distracting details; show unfamiliar subjects; or familiar objects shown from an unusual view. Another reason for misunderstanding is when too much information is presented and people cannot absorb it all. More information on visual perception is given later in this chapter.

Stage 4: promoting change (acceptance)

A communication should not only be received and understood – it should be believed and accepted. In Chapter 2 some of the reasons why a particular belief might be difficult to change were discussed. It is easier to change beliefs when they have been acquired only recently. It is more difficult to influence a belief that has been held for a long time or if people already have well-developed beliefs on the topic (which is often the case). It is usually easier to promote a belief when its effects can be easily demonstrated, e.g. that ventilated improved pit latrines do not smell. If a belief is held by the whole community, or is part of a wider belief system such as their religion, we can predict that it will be very difficult to change by methods such as mass media and leaflets.

Later in this chapter you will see how the nature of the source and content of the message can influence whether people believe and accept the message.

Stage 5: producing a change in behaviour

A communication may result in a change in beliefs and attitude but still not influence behaviour. This can happen when the communication has not been targeted at the belief that has the most influence on the person's attitude to the behaviour. For example, many communication programmes have emphasised the dangers of diarrhoea and failed to give enough emphasis on dehydration.

A person may have a favourable attitude and want to carry out the action, e.g. use family planning, bring the child for immunisation etc. However, pressure from other people in the family or community may prevent the person from doing it.

Another reason a person may not perform a behaviour is a lack of enabling factors such as money, time, skills or health services. The role of culture, beliefs, social pressure and enabling factors are discussed in detail in the previous chapter.

Stage 6: improvement in health

Improvements in health will only take place if the behaviours have been carefully selected so that they really do influence health. If your messages are based on out-dated and incorrect ideas, people could follow our advice but their health will not improve. This need to ensure accurate advice was the reason why *The Facts for Life* initiative was launched by UNICEF, WHO and UNESCO (see page 8).

Components of communications

In looking at the factors which influence success of a communication, it is helpful to consider separately and distinguish between the *receiver, source, message* and *channel*.

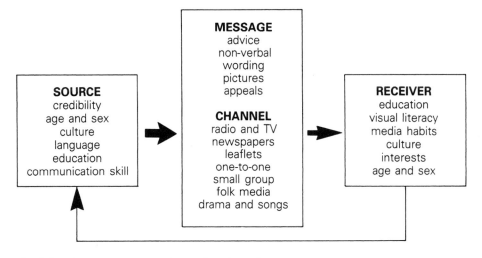

Fig. 3.3   Source, message, channel and receiver

Receiver (audience)

The first step in planning any communication is to consider the intended audience. A method that will be effective with one audience may not succeed with another. Two people may hear the same radio programme, see the same poster or attend the same talk and interpret them quite differently. Some of the main information you need to find out when planning communications are shown in Figure 3.4. You should also refer to the list of questions about patterns of influence and health beliefs on pages 31 and 34.

Source

People are exposed to communications from many different sources and are more likely to believe a communication from a person or organisation that they trust, i.e. has high source credibility. Think about the communities you are familiar with and ask yourself: what special qualities makes a person trusted? What can make the community lose trust in a person?

In considering these questions you can refer to the discussion of opinion leaders, significant others and social pressure in the previous chapter and the detailed check list of questions on page 31. Rural persons are not usually impressed by educational status and have more

regard for personal qualities. People do not believe radio programmes or posters just because they are produced by the Ministry of Health. The health education worker is often not the most credible source. You will need to find out who your intended audience respect and involve these opinion leaders in your health education. Depending on the community, trust and *source-credibility* may come from:

- a person's natural position in the family community, e.g. village chief or elder;
- through their personal qualities or actions, e.g. a health worker who always comes out to help people even at night;
- qualifications and training;
- the extent to which the source shares characteristics such as age, culture, education, experiences with the receiver.

In which of the cases in Figure 3.5 do you think that communication will be more effective? A person from a similar background to the community is more likely to share the same language, ideas and motivations and thus be a more effective communicator. One of the main reasons for communication failure is when the source comes from a different background from the receiver and uses inappropriate message content and appeals.

This principle – that people who share similar backgrounds communicate better with

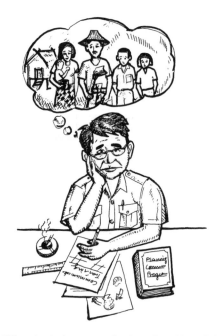

Educational factors. What is their age and educational level? What kinds of
arguments and appeals might convince them? Can they read? What words do they
use in their everyday conversation? Are they used to looking at pictures and diagrams?
Socio-cultural factors. What do they already know, believe and feel about the topic
of the communication? How strongly-held are their present beliefs? What values do
they hold to be important? Whose opinions and views do they trust? How open are
they to new ideas?
Pattern of communication. What patterns of communication already exist in the
community? Are there any rules surrounding the discussion of health topics openly?
What rules are there for conversation between people? How do people show respect
when talking to another person? Where do people find out about health issues? Do
they listen to the radio or television? What time of day and which programmes do
they listen to? Which, if any, books, newspapers or magazines do they read? Do
people put up pictures or calendars in their homes? What traditional media such as
songs or drama do they enjoy? Which places do they pass that might be good places
to put up posters?

Fig. 3.4   Questions to ask about your audience for planning communication

each other – has important implications for
health education. It explains why health
workers who are strangers to the local community are not always effective in their health
education work. Because of this, many health
education programmes recruit field agents and
volunteers from the community in which they
are serving.

Even if the field workers do not come from
the local community, it is still possible to help
them become closer to the community. The
word *empathy* is used to describe the process by
which a person learns to understand how others
feel and think. Empathy is essential to becoming
a good communicator. An important part of
communication skill training is helping people
to develop empathy with their communities.
The best way to develop empathy is role-play
which is described in Chapter 4. In role-play,
you can try out situations and learn what it feels
like to be a member of the community, such as
a mother having to find time to prepare oral
rehydration therapy or to overcome opposition
from the grandmother.

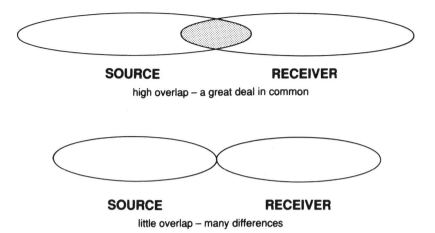

SOURCE   **RECEIVER**

high overlap – a great deal in common

SOURCE   **RECEIVER**

little overlap – many differences

Fig. 3.5   Source and receiver in communication

The communication message

The message consists of what is actually communicated including the actual appeals, words, pictures and sounds that you use to get the ideas across.

The nature of the advice given

A message will only be effective if the advice presented is relevant, appropriate, acceptable and put across in an understandable way. In deciding what advice to give, you will need to apply both an understanding of health and disease as well as the various influences on behaviour described in the previous chapter.

The type of appeal

The appeal is the way we organise the content of the message to persuade or convince people.

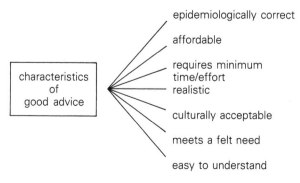

Fig. 3.6   Characteristics of good advice

There is a tendency for many health communications to use logical arguments that rely heavily on medical details. However, many other approaches are possible.

Types of appeals in health communications

Fear – a message may try to frighten people into action by emphasising the serious outcome from not taking action. Symbols such as dying persons, coffins, grave stones, skulls may be used.

Humour – the message is conveyed in a funny way such as a cartoon.

Logical/factual appeal – emphasis in the message on conveying the need for action by giving of facts, figures and information, e.g. on the causes of disease.

Emotional appeal – attempts to convince people by arousing emotions, images and feelings rather than giving facts and figures, e.g. showing smiling babies, wealthy families with latrines etc., associating the action with sex.

One-sided message – only presents the advantages of taking action and does not mention any possible disadvantages.

Two-sided message – presents both the benefits and disadvantages ('pros and cons') of taking action.

Positive appeals – communications that ask people to do something, e.g. breastfeed your child, build a latrine.

Negative appeals – communications that ask people NOT to do something – i.e. do not bottle-feed your child, do not defecate in the bush.

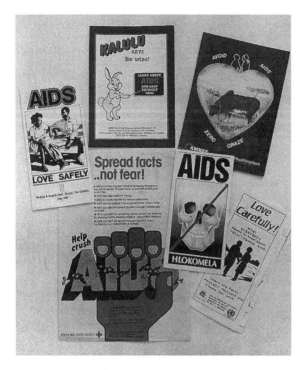

Fig. 3.7   Examples of appeals

Not everyone responds in the same way to a message. What might convince you might be quite different from what might persuade another person. For example what kinds of appeals do you think might convince each of the following: persons with little schooling; persons of a high educational level; children; and health workers?

Fear appeal. Evidence suggests that mild fear can arouse interest, create concern and lead to change. However, too much fear can lead to people denying and rejecting the message. For example, health education on smoking in Britain used fear approaches of showing diseased lungs and descriptions of the harmful effects of smoking. This had little effect on smokers who built up a barrier of beliefs to deny the message and justify their smoking. Education on AIDS in many countries has involved fear appeals including symbols of death such as skulls. With some people this has resulted in laughter and failure to take seriously the risk of AIDS; with others this approach has led to panic responses, stress and anxiety.

However, the use of fear is not simply a case of whether it will persuade people to act. It involves ethical issues as well. Fear might be aroused but a person may not be able to take action to change – this can lead to considerable stress and anxiety. Many health educators feel that it is wrong to try and frighten people into action – unless there is clear evidence that benefits in health would result and that the means (i.e. enabling factors) are readily available to perform the action.

Humour. Humour is a very good way of attracting interest and attention. It can also serve a useful role to lighten the tension when dealing with serious subjects. Enjoyment and entertainment can result in highly effective remembering and learning. However, humour does not always lead to changes in beliefs and attitudes. Humour is also very subjective – what one person finds funny another person may not.

Logical/factual compared with emotional appeals. A repeated observation from health education programmes throughout the world is that information on its own is usually not enough to change beliefs, attitudes and behaviour. Logical factual arguments discussing disease patterns, parasite cycles and epidemiology will only carry weight with persons of a high educational level. Persons with less education will often be more convinced by simple emotional appeals from people they trust and stressing locally-held values such as motherhood, prestige, strength, etc.

Despite this, many health educators still feel that it is important to present some factual information because it allows people to make informed decisions. But it is important to be realistic about the limitations of just relying on facts to persuade people.

One-sided compared with two-sided messages. Presenting only one side of an argument may be effective if your audience will not be exposed to different views. However, if they are likely to hear opposing information, it can create suspicion that you are hiding something and not being honest. If there are some drawbacks to taking your advice – such as side effects from a drug – it is better to be honest and admit them rather than let people find them out for themselves and then blame you for concealing them. Many health educators would also say that their main emphasis is not just to make people change behaviour but to help communities develop decision-making and problem-solving skills. Giving different points of view and helping them to distinguish the best actions to take is an important part of this process.

When you are face-to-face with individuals or groups it is easy to present both sides and make sure that the audience understands the issues. This is much more difficult in mass media such as radio, television and newspapers where the audience may only grasp part of the message or selectively pick up the points that they agree with. If you present both sides on the mass media you must test these messages carefully to make sure that the audience is not confused by receiving different points of view.

Positive and negative appeals. Negative appeals use terms such as 'avoid...' or 'don't...' to discourage people from performing harmful behaviours, e.g. 'don't bottle-feed', 'do not defecate in the bush'. Most health educators agree that it is better to be positive and promote a beneficial behaviour, e.g. 'breastfeed your baby', 'use a latrine'.

Formats

In theory, a message could use any of the five senses: sight, hearing, touch, taste and smell. However, the senses we mainly use in health communications are hearing and sight.

A great deal of information can be conveyed through sounds. Words can either be in spoken or written form and as songs. In addition to words, much information is conveyed through *non-verbal communication.* This includes gestures, hand movements, direction of looking, tone of voice and appearance. A more detailed discussion of the important role that non-verbal communication plays in face-to-face communication is provided in Chapter 5.

In a book, information is conveyed in both the pictures and the words. You can use more than one format at a time: for example a health worker talking to a person and showing a leaflet or flip-chart would involve formats for face-to-face and leaflets described in Table 3.2.

Table 3.2 Formats used in different communication methods

Face-to-face	spoken words non-verbal communication visual – real objects and models pictures/written words (when a visual aid is used)
Mass media	
radio	spoken words, non-verbal communication
television	spoken words, visual format non-verbal communication, written words
leaflets, books, newspapers	written words, visual pictures

Actual content of message

This includes the actual words, pictures, sounds that make up the communication and convey the appeals. In a radio programme the content would be a mix of: the advice given, wording, tone of voice, music. A poster would contain the basic appeal, pictures, words, photographs, symbols and colours.

In visual communications we can carry out a 'visual analysis' and analyse the content of a visual communication and specify:

- what is actually said; which words are used;
- the type of letters used; whether capital letters (UPPER CASE) or small letters (lower case), lettering style, e.g. ordinary, *italics* or **bold**;
- size of the actual letters;
- colour and printing method;
- the pictures used (illustrations), whether photographs (with or without backgrounds), or drawings (detailed, simple line drawings, or stylised drawings/cartoons);
- the size and colour of the pictures.

How does the message influence attention?

Decisions such as whether to listen to one radio programme or another are deliberate ones. But others take place without conscious thought such as whether we happen to notice one poster out of many when we are going down a street or choose a particular book on a shelf.

A good example of the brain's ability to select information is the 'cocktail party phenomenon'. In a crowded room you can concentrate on listening to the person you are talking with and filter out the noise of all the other persons. But your ears and brain are still receiving all the other noises and if someone mentions something significant such as your own name you will notice – pay attention to – it.

It has been suggested by the psychologist Broadbent that the human brain acts as a filter (Figure 3.8). The brain processes the information it receives from the senses and decides what it will ignore and what it will pay attention to and interpret.

Think about what communications have attracted your attention recently and see if you can draw any lessons. What characteristics would draw your attention to each of the following: a magazine on a magazine stall; a radio programme; a poster on a wall with other posters? The factors that make communications attract attention fall into two main groups: physical and motivational characteristics.

Physical characteristics that attract attention include:

- size, e.g. of the whole poster – we are more likely to notice a large poster or book than a small one; size of letters – large letters on a poster, title words;
- intensity – bold headings in a sentence, poster;
- high pitched sounds, baby crying, police sirens, loud noises;
- colour – primary colours such as reds, yellows, orange;
- pictures – pictures and drawings.

Motivational characteristics that attract attention include:

- novelty – unusual features, unfamiliar and surprising objects;
- interest – interests/felt needs of audience and perceived relevance to audience – people look at things they are interested in and want to know something about;
- deeper motivations – appeals to motivations and drives of audience, e.g. sex;
- entertainment and humour.

The design of a poster, including colour, size, lettering and use of pictures can increase its likelihood of gaining attention and being noticed. Communications that attract attention are also those which deal with subjects that the target group *want* to know something about, i.e. fit in with their felt needs and interests. Another way of attracting attention is by including something unusual in the communication to arouse interest. You can include unusual objects in exhibitions, incorporate drama in a public meeting, have an unusual picture on a poster, begin a radio programme with an attention-getting sound.

Many health communications have failed because they have been boring, dull and emphasise medical facts. You should remember that people like to be entertained – and that, just because you are interested in the subject, it does not mean that others will be. You should explore ways of making your educational work interesting and fun. For example, if you are making a radio programme you can make it more interesting by using a variety of formats including music, drama, interviews, quizzes etc.

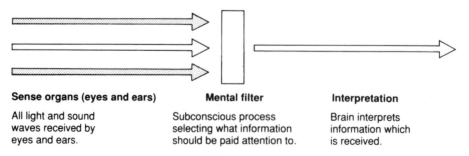

Sense organs (eyes and ears)	Mental filter	Interpretation
All light and sound waves received by eyes and ears.	Subconscious process selecting what information should be paid attention to.	Brain interprets information which is received.

Fig. 3.8 Broadbent Filter Model of selective attention

You can read more about entertainment and media in Chapters 7 and 8.

It is also important to hold attention in face-to-face communication and teaching sessions so your audience listens carefully. In the next chapter you will see how an important function of learning aids is to arouse the interest of a group.

Perception and understanding

Problems in understanding take place when the person receiving the message misinterprets the various words, pictures and non-verbal signals that make up the message. It is not difficult to understand how misunderstandings take place when the message is in an unfamiliar language. It is also obvious that the writing in a leaflet or poster will not be understood by a person who cannot read and write. However, even when persons speak the same language, there can be problems in communication – for example if unfamiliar or technical words are used. It is also easy to come to the wrong conclusions about the meaning of looks, gestures and tones of voice that make up non-verbal communication.

Because of the need to communicate to illiterate persons, health educators often put emphasis on using pictures rather than words in posters and leaflets. It was thought that pictures are a universal language. However pictures themselves contain a 'visual language' with special ways for showing distance, direction, motion and even emotions such as happiness and strength.

A picture is drawn on a flat sheet of paper but the real world is solid. A picture can only show one part of an object whereas in the real world we can walk around an object to see many different views. Drawings usually simplify objects and have less detail. The real world is in colour whereas the high expense of colour printing means that pictures in books are often in black and white. People who have not had much experience of looking at pictures can easily misinterpret the message. *Visual literacy* is the term used for a person's familiarity with pictures.

Some of the well-known studies of visual literacy have been carried out in Kenya, Nepal, Lesotho, Zambia and Ghana. These have involved showing a range of pictures to samples of the community to find out which ones they could correctly identify. Some of the kinds of pictures that were not understood include: stylised diagrams, e.g. line drawings, 'stick men', silhouettes and use of shading to show light and shadows; biological diagrams such as life cycles, pictures of organs, anatomical drawings, parts of body; pictures showing emotions such as happiness, strength and sickness; pictures using artist's conventions for showing movement, relative size of objects, as well as relative distances (horizons, converging lines etc.); symbols such as +, −, ×, %, √, →; using of colours to show feelings, e.g. red for danger. Some examples of different pictures used in these studies are shown in Figure 3.9.

These visual literacy studies tell us a great deal about the psychological processes involved in perception. When people hear or see something they try to give it a meaning that 'makes sense' to them. Perception thus involves *guessing* at the meaning from the information available. If not enough information is available in a picture, the guess may be wrong and the picture not understood. In radio programmes there is often the background noises of other programmes, which can make it difficult to make out the words. A similar problem can be found in pictures when there is too much information, distracting backgrounds and unnecessary details.

Perception does not happen instantly but is a process over a short time period (see Figure 3.10). A person will take in the different information (or 'clues') and arrive at an interpretation. We can even measure this with machines that follow eye movements. A person will first look at the striking or unusual features that attract attention and then take in further details until the interpretation is reached. In trying to guess the meaning of a part of a picture, a person will take into account the background. If the picture is not immediately obvious, the person will choose an interpretation that fits with the details that caught his/her attention in the background.

Perception depends on a person's experience. You will find difficulty recognising and giving a

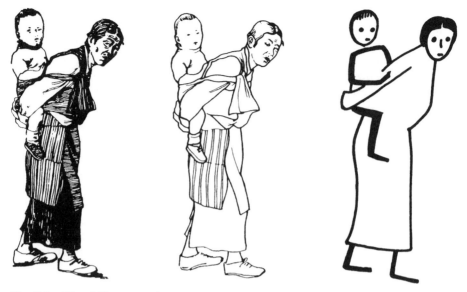

Fig. 3.9   Visual literacy styles

name to something that you have never seen before. For example, a study in Kenya found that a person seeing a picture of a cupboard who has never seen a real cupboard before was not able to identify it and instead identified it as something else.

Problems of misunderstanding can be particularly serious with mass media with its lack of immediate feedback to check if correct understanding has taken place. Misunderstandings of communications are more likely to take place when the artist, radio producer or communication designer comes from a different background from that of the target audience. This is espe-

cially so when the audience is rural and of low educational status and the communication planners are urban, highly educated and from different cultural backgrounds. The best way of overcoming this cultural distance between the communication planners and the community is to find ways of involving the community in the production of the materials. It is also important to pre-test the prototypes (first versions) carefully before they are broadcast or printed.

As education and access to printed materials increases, so also should people become more familiar with interpreting pictures. A study by UNICEF in Nepal, *Rethinking Visual Literacy*,

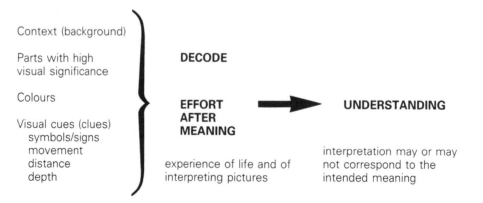

Fig. 3.10   The process of visual perception

showed that, with a small teaching input, it is not difficult to learn to understand pictures. I have summarised the findings of a number studies on visual communication to produce the guidelines on p. 60.

Even with these guidelines it is essential to *pre-test* any communication that is used. Pre-testing involves showing draft ('proto-type') versions of the materials to individuals and groups of the intended audience and checking for understanding, acceptability and appropriateness by asking the questions on p. 60. The example given is that for a poster or leaflet but similar questions could be asked when pre-testing radio and television programmes and advertisements.

Channel

This is also sometimes referred to as the *communication method*. There are two main groups of methods: face-to-face ('interpersonal') and mass media. Each channel provides opportunities to use a different combination of *formats* (see Table 3.3).

Mass media include broadcast media (radio and television) as well as print media (newspapers, books, leaflets and wall posters) and these are described in more detail in Chapter 8. Television involves both a sound and visual dimension. Radio involves sound only. Radio ownership is high in many countries, which makes it a particularly valuable medium where the literacy rate is low. Print media such as newspapers, books and leaflets use the written word, as well as requiring an ability to understand pictures, so are only appropriate for audiences who can read.

Face-to-face or interpersonal methods of communication include all those forms involving direct interaction between the source and receiver. Examples of face-to-face methods with increasing audience size are: one-to-one and counselling; small group (fewer than 12 persons); intermediate group/lecture (between 12 and 30 people); and large group lecture /public meeting (more than 30 people). The main advantage of face-to-face communication over mass media is that it creates opportunities for questions, discussion, participation and feedback. It is possible to check that you have been

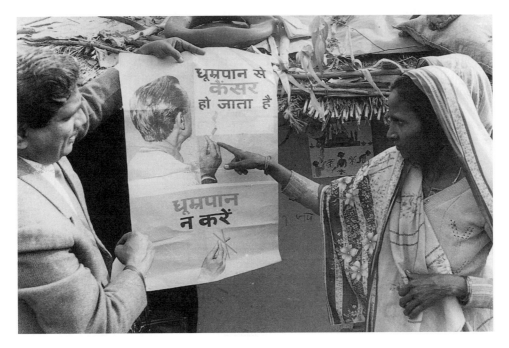

Fig. 3.11   Pre-testing posters in India

Guidelines to using pictures	Questions to ask when pre-testing materials
1. Make details accurate and of objects familiar to the target audience. 2. Avoid distracting details. 3. If you use colour make it accurate. 4. Distortions in size (e.g. enlargements) should be avoided. 5. Show complete objects – especially parts of the body. 6. Show objects from familiar angles (be careful of cross-sections and anatomical drawings). 7. Be careful when using perspective (showing relative distance). 8. Use signs and symbols that are understood by the target audience. 9. Be careful when using sequences of pictures as it can easily cause confusion. 10. Single communications should not contain more than one message. 11. Always pre-test with samples of your intended audience.	Please read back the words and explain what the words and pictures mean to you? What is the message that you think this communication is trying to get across? Is there anything that you think is not clear? Is there anything that you do not like and offends you? How relevant is the message to you? Do you think that you would put the advice into practice yourself? If not, why not? What additional information do you think should be provided? How do you think it could be improved?

understood and give further explanations. However, as the size of the group increases, it is more difficult to have feedback and discussion. In large groups and public meetings only a small number usually take part and many persons feel shy speaking out. Public meetings thus share many the characteristics of mass media in that they involve limited participation and feedback.

We can look at the direction of flow of communication in community settings. At the beginning of this chapter and in the previous chapter you saw how it was important to consider sources of influence and 'opinion leadership' in families and communities. You can represent the communication pattern or 'social network' in a community by a diagram such as Figure 3.12. The lines represent a line of communication between two people.

Analysing the flow of communication in a community ('sociometric' analysis) will show if there are 'opinion leaders'. They may be elders, shopkeepers or just people who have acquired some influence or importance. They form the *internal communication system* within a community that you need to understand before planning any health education activities. If you can obtain the full support of the opinion leaders then it should be easy to convince a community to take up health-promoting innovations. If the opinion

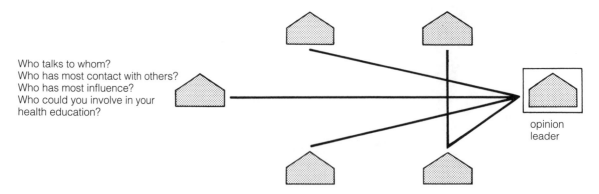

Who talks to whom?
Who has most contact with others?
Who has most influence?
Who could you involve in your health education?

opinion leader

Fig. 3.12   Communication networks in communities

leaders are against you it will be extremely difficult to work in a community.

The expansion of printed media, radio and television that is taking place makes it easy to forget that most traditional forms of communication involve face-to-face or *oral communication*. Traditional or 'popular' media such as drama, singing, dancing, story telling and proverb telling may exist in your community. Community gatherings, religious meetings, ceremonies can provide opportunities for health education. This provides an example of the approach of 'starting where people are at' rather than imposing forms of communication that are unfamiliar to the community. Chapter 7 describes how you can mobilise popular media for health education and health promotion.

Comparison of mass media and face-to-face communication methods

Mass media are the best methods for rapid spread of simple information and facts to a large population at low cost. If the advice is realistic (see Figure 3.6) and the message pre-tested, the message can be accurately transmitted without the distortions that can sometimes take place when we rely on word of mouth.

However, as mass media are broadcast to the whole population, they are not a good method for selectively reaching specific groups, e.g. grandmothers or teenagers. It is difficult to make the message appropriate to the special situation of local communities whose problems and needs may be different from the rest of the country. Even if a person hears something on the radio and wishes to change, he or she may be pressurised against change by those around them. Furthermore, health education often involves influencing beliefs and attitudes and developing problem-solving skills. For these more difficult objectives, participatory learning methods involving group discussion, sharing of experience and problem-solving exercises will be more effective.

Face-to-face methods are slower for spreading information in a population because of the need to mobilise fieldworkers and travel to the different communities to hold meetings. However, the opportunity to ask the audience questions and obtain feedback gives face-to-face methods a powerful advantage. It is possible to contact specific groups, make the advice relevant to their special needs and develop problem-solving skills and community participation. Feedback makes it possible to check for misunderstandings and give clarification and explain particular points.

The communications researcher Everett Rogers has reviewed many studies of how new practices or 'innovations' spread or 'diffuse' within communities. He suggests that adoption of new practices such as using latrines or oral rehydration therapy takes place through stages: initially a person becomes aware of the existence of the new practice; he/she may become interested, then decide to try it out and, if

Table 3.3 Main characteristics of mass media and face-to-face channels

Characteristics	Mass media	Face-to-face
speed to cover large population	rapid	slow
accuracy and lack of distortion	high accuracy	easily distorted
ability to select particular audience	difficult to select audience	can be highly selective
direction	one-way	two-way
ability to respond to local needs of specific communities	only provides non-specific information	can fit to local need
feed-back	only indirect feedback from surveys	direct feedback possible
main effect	increased/knowledge awareness	changes in attitudes and behaviour; problem-solving skills

awareness   ←   mass media
↓
interest
↓
trial   ←   face-to-face
↓
adoption

Fig. 3.13   Influence of communication methods on adoption of innovations

satisfied, adopt it. Rogers' *Communication of Innovations Theory* suggests that mass media can provide the necessary background information for change but are usually insufficient on their own to change behaviour – especially if you are

trying to change long-established customs. Most health behaviour changes will require face-to-face communication using community-based approaches, home visiting, involvement of opinion leaders and community participation.

Mostly, it is not simply a case of either mass media or interpersonal methods. A well-planned programme will involve a carefully chosen *mix* of both approaches which exploits their different advantages. Figure 3.14 shows a communication strategy for an oral rehydration programme in Honduras. This combined different approaches with activities timed to coincide with the seasonal peaks in diarrhoea. Radio reinforces the face-to-face communication by field workers and printed materials have been produced to support the programme.

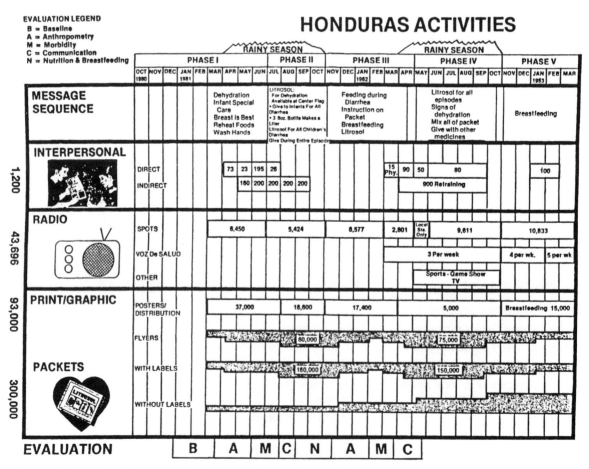

Fig. 3.14   Communication strategy for promotion of oral rehydration in Honduras

Deciding what communication method to use

Choice of communication method and supporting learning aids will depend on what you are trying to achieve, the nature of your audience and what resources are at your disposal (Figure 3.15). Some of the questions you will need to ask to make this decision are listed below. The starting point for selection of media should be your analysis of what you are trying to convey. Are you going to try to change a belief – and will it be a weakly held one or a strongly held one rooted in culture or experience as described in the previous chapter? What type of learning will you be trying to promote? You should read the section on learning in the next chapter, which will show how you can separate out the learning involved into simple and complex facts, skills and attitudes.

Each method provides different opportunities for formats including visual, sounds, verbal and non-verbal communication (see Table 3.2). If you want to help a person to recognise a child's fast breathing at the onset of a severe respiratory infection you will need a medium with the dimension of sound. If you want to show someone what a condom or an improved latrine *looks* like, you will need a method that has a visual dimension.

In addition, you will also have to consider practical considerations of cost, complexity and feasibility of use. If you are working in a local community you are unlikely to have access to mass media such as radio or newspapers. You may not have any fieldworkers at your disposal so have no choice but to concentrate on methods that do not require staffing.

A useful guide to planning your health education is to start with simpler methods first, such as radio, leaflets and posters and see if they are effective. Only if the simple methods do not work should you move on to more expensive methods involving extensive use of fieldworkers and other interpersonal methods. Short-term approaches can be accompanied by longer-term strategies such as working through schools and the workplace.

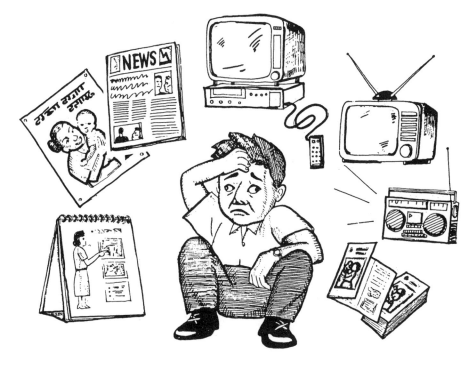

Fig. 3.15   Choice of methods

Criteria for selecting methods

Your 'learning' objectives
Do you need to convey simple facts, complex information, problem-solving skills, practical manual ('psycho-motor') skills, attitudes and behaviour change? (See Chapter 4 for further discussion of learning.)

Other programme considerations
Will you need a visual dimension, e.g. picture to explain your point? Is sound necessary?
How accepting is the community of new ideas?
Will there be resistance your advice?
How urgent is your timescale? Is it a short- or long-term priority?
Do you want to develop community participation?

Characteristics of the audience
What are the characteristics of the audience that will affect choice of methods? e.g. age, experience of life, education and literacy level, previous exposure to pictures; ownership of radio/TVs, listening, watching and reading habits; familiarity with different media, traditional communication methods already in use? (See also audience characteristics on page 52, Figure 3.4)

Characteristics of different methods
How much will the different methods cost including initial costs and operating and maintenance?
How many staff and what level of skill is involved in using the method?
What field requirements will affect the use of the equipment, e.g. for electricity, blackout, storage and transport?

Costs
Are funds available for initial purchase, spare parts and maintenance?
Will you need electricity or a black-out?
What will be the need for need for trained staff for media production, maintenance and implementation?
Will you need trained fieldworkers in the community to implement the method?

Case studies of planned communication activities to promote health (see also the case studies in other chapters on use of mass media, folk media and face-to-face communication)

Promoting immunisation in an urban community in Cape Town South Africa.
Community health workers, student nurses and health inspectors carried out a 3-week intensive campaign using community leaders and used two mobile units equipped with loud hailers, stickers, pamphlets, posters, radio, and newspapers. Immunisation coverage increased from 56% before the campaign to 71% afterwards.

Mass media and interpersonal health education on acute respiratory infection (ARI) in Malaysia.
Health workers were trained on case management of ARI. A mobile health education team travelled to the villages giving talks on ARI control and leaflets were distributed to households. Billboards showing key messages were placed at markets and other locations. Mothers attending well-baby clinics were shown a video followed by health education talks on recognition of symptoms and signs of pneumonia and its management. An evaluation found a significant reduction in severe ARI cases in the intervention community compared with a similar area that only received routine education.

Promoting birth spacing among the Maya-Quiché of Guatemala.
A 3-year communication campaign was combined with training of health workers, improving contraceptive supply and recruiting volunteer promoters. The communication component consisted of a generalised TV campaign at the whole population and a targeted campaign directed at the illiterate Mayan community, which included: two radio spots, a vehicle-mounted loudspeaker playing messages at markets and other community settings and a video produced in the local language for showing to meetings and triggering discussions. An evaluation found increases in both knowledge and use of contraception over the 3-year period.

Evaluation of printed materials for promoting breastfeeding in South Africa. Pictures were prepared by an artist to support 10-minute talks by nurses to illiterate mothers at antenatal clinics. Key messages were (1) breastfeeding creates a stronger bond between mother and baby than does bottle-feeding; and (2) clean water, sterilised bottles, and correct formula mixture all directly affect the health of bottle-fed babies. A follow-up questionnaire to 47 mothers found that only 9% of the mothers could identify the black and white illustrations but 65% could identify colour pictures.

AIDS education using advertisements on buses in Johannesburg, South Africa. A 6-month campaign with ads on the back of 30 buses stating: 'Learn about AIDS and keep yourself safe. Phone 339–2345. JHB City Health Dept.' This message was selected from a list of ten possibilities by telephoning 52 random adults. It was estimated that a minimum of 57,970 persons saw the messages. However, only 229 persons telephoned the Health Department on the number provided, which was a disappointing result.

Summary

Communication planning involves two main groups of decisions: what are the aims of the communication and who should be the target group? Making these decisions involves the application of ideas introduced in the first two chapters concerned with health education, health promotion and influences on behaviour.

The second set of decisions has been the subject of this chapter – the choice of source, messages and channels required to promote the desired changes.

1 A communication can go through a series of stages before it can have an impact on the improvement of health. These stages are: reaching the senses; gaining attention; understanding; acceptance of the message; and change in behaviour. A detailed understanding of the characteristics of the community is needed to make decisions about the best source, message and channel.

2 Messages should be pre-tested to make sure that they will attract attention, be correctly understood, acceptable and relevant to the problem. This is especially important with mass media when the message has to stand on its own and there's no opportunity to check for misunderstanding.

3 Communication should be evaluated to find out if it has achieved each of the six stages from reaching the senses to improvement of health. Lessons learnt from evaluation should be used to design better programmes.

4 Conclusions from the Chapter 3 can be combined with the basic principles of communication theory introduced in this chapter to produce the guidelines for effective health communications listed here.

Characteristics of effective health communications

Promotes actions that are realistic and feasible within the constraints faced by the community.
Builds on ideas, concepts and practices that people already have.
Repeated and reinforced over time using different methods.
Adaptable, and uses existing channels of communication – for example songs, drama and storytelling.
Entertaining and attracts community's attention.
Uses clear simple language with local expressions and emphasises short-term benefits of action.
Provides opportunities for dialogue and discussion to allow learner participation and feedback on understanding and implementation.
Uses demonstrations to show the benefits of adopting practices.

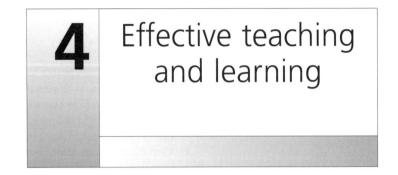

4 Effective teaching and learning

If I only hear it, I forget it.
When people just sit and listen to someone else talk, they will not learn very much.

If I hear and see it, I remember it.
When people see for themselves what things look like and how they work, they will learn more than if they just listened to someone else talk about it.

If I hear, see and do it, I know it.
When people not only hear and see, but actually do, make and discover things for themselves, they will learn the most.

Teaching and learning are essential to most health education and health promotion activities. Training is really another word for teaching. It is often applied to the process of introducing fieldworkers to new ideas, information and skills – either in their initial training or later as part of their *continuing* education.

People can learn in many different ways. This chapter will deal with learning that takes place through organised face-to-face situations in groups – either small or large. It will build on concepts of communication introduced in the previous chapter as well as set the scene for the discussion of face-to-face communication in the next chapter. It will help you to:

1 Decide what to include in your teaching – i.e. set the objectives.
2 Choose teaching methods and learning aids.
3 Plan training courses.

Deciding what to include in your teaching

You may only have a few hours available with a particular group, or as much as a month. In either case you will have to decide what are the most important topics to cover, and set priority objectives for your teaching. Objectives are precise statements of what you intend to achieve through your planned learning activities. Setting objectives will help you to decide: what to include in the learning activities; what learning methods to use and; how to assess the effectiveness of your teaching activities. A *curriculum* is a set of objectives with details of the learning methods by which you will reach those objectives.

The initial reason for planning some teaching is usually a need that has arisen in your work. For example, you may have to update field workers on a new disease such as AIDS, introduce new skills such as preparation of oral rehydration solution or preparation and use of a learning aid such as flip charts.

In planning training we begin by specifying the behaviours – sometimes called 'competencies' – that the fieldworkers must be able to perform in order to contribute to the health education programme. This list of desired actions is often called a *job description* or *job specification* and forms the basis of identifying training needs, e.g. Figure 4.1. Preparing a job

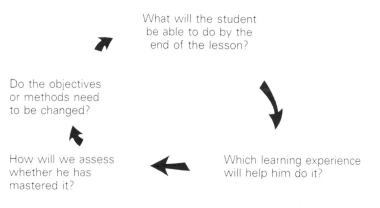

What will the student be able to do by the end of the lesson?

Do the objectives or methods need to be changed?

How will we assess whether he has mastered it?

Which learning experience will help him do it?

Fig. 4.1 Curriculum design and objective setting for training programmes

description and resulting curriculum involves asking the questions in Figure 4.2.

You can prepare a job description by: studying the problem and possible solutions; observing successful fieldworkers and the methods they have used; consulting other persons with relevant experience. Your proposed job description should be realistic and feasible.

Many fieldworkers already have job descriptions that form the basis for their conditions of employment. The job specification that you develop for planning a training programme will

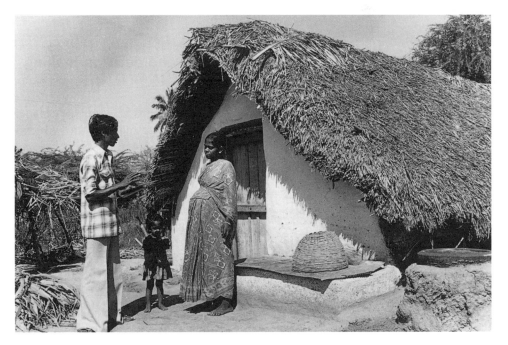

- What do you require the community or fieldworker to *do* to implement the programme you have planned? These actions should be written out as a detailed job specification.
- What activities in the job specification is the person already able to undertake?
- What activities in the job specification will the person require training to be able to undertake?
- What does the person require to learn to carry out those activities?

Fig. 4.2 Questions to ask in preparing a job specification

usually be more detailed. It should describe the kinds of decisions and educational methods the person will be expected to use in their work. You can then evaluate the training by finding out whether, at the end of the teaching programme, the participants can actually undertake the activities you have specified. (In the final chapter, you will also see that decisions about job specifications for key fieldworkers form an important part of the process of programme planning.)

Sample job specification of the health education duties of a rural health assistant

1. Carry out a community diagnosis to determine: health education needs; influences on behaviour; opinion leaders and social networks.
2. Carry out one-to-one health education with a range of persons on topics such as water supply, sanitation, food hygiene and nutrition.
3. Carry out group health education with community groups.
4. Give health education talks at public meetings.
5. Advise teachers on school health education and give talks to pupils in classes.
6. Advise families on setting up kitchen gardens for promotion of nutrition.
7. Supervise health education activities of community health workers.
8. Prepare health education demonstration programmes on water supply and sanitation.
9. Work as a part of a team with other personnel in the promotion of primary health care and integrated rural development.
10. Collect local data for planning and evaluating health education programmes.

Task analysis and specifying the kinds of learning

The kinds of learning involving intellectual or thinking tasks are called 'cognitive' learning. These are distinguished from 'affective' learning which covers emotions, feelings, attitudes and values. The different kinds of learning include:

- *knowledge* facts, specific information;
- *skills*
  ○ 'thinking' decision-making and problem-solving skills;
  ○ communication skills, e.g. one-to-one and group;
  ○ psychomotor skills, e.g. handling, mixing;
- *attitudes* feelings, emotions, values.

The word 'know' is used in a vague way in everyday speech. Consider the following: knowing the life cycle of hookworm, knowing how to design a sanitation programme, knowing how to build a latrine and knowing how to talk to a community meeting. These are each quite different kinds of learning and are respectively: factual knowledge, decision-making skills, psychomotor skills and communication skills.

Each activity in a job description will require a different combination of knowledge, skills, and attitudes. The term *task analysis* is used for the process of analysing the actions in a job description to determine the kinds of learning involved.

Knowledge and decision-making skills

A useful way of separating types of cognitive learning was suggested by the educationist Bloom. He suggests that there are different levels of cognitive learning. These range from simpler 'lower-order' cognitive skills, such as factual knowledge and comprehension, to more complex 'higher-order' skills, such as application, analysis, synthesis and evaluation, which can be called problem-solving skills.

Knowledge is the simplest level and includes knowledge of terms, facts and principles. Examples are:

- listing the causes of diarrhoea,
- describing the ways in which diarrhoea can be prevented,
- describing how bacteria can cause infection.

Some facts can be simple to learn. Others, such as the life cycle of a parasite are more difficult, especially if it is an unfamiliar subject. Teaching facts involves the following steps:

relating the information to previous knowledge; presenting the information logically in a step-by-step fashion; using visual aids to explain relationships and avoiding presenting too much information in one session and causing overload. Face-to-face contact is helpful for explaining more complicated facts as it is possible to ask questions to check understanding. If the facts are simple and the educational level of your audience is sufficiently high, you can use distance learning methods such as a newsletter or books.

More complex *'higher order'* thinking skills involve application of knowledge, interpretation of facts, theories, problem-solving and decision-making; these usually require some knowledge first. Some examples of thinking skills are given below, with more difficult higher order ones given at the end of the list:

- interpretation of facts, relationships or theories;
- separating preventive behaviours into primary, secondary and tertiary;
- interpretation of existing data, such as determining the health problems of communities from clinic data;
- choosing a balanced diet from the foods provided;
- using a growth chart to assess whether an infant is at risk of developing malnutrition;
- analysing the influences on a person's health behaviour;
- writing a radio script to encourage mothers to breastfeed;
- designing an educational programme for the prevention of diarrhoea;
- deriving a theory to explain relationships, e.g. construction of a model to explain why people do not use health services;
- evaluation of a health education plan for the promotion of breastfeeding.

Decision-making skills are taught by: first providing the necessary basic information; then demonstrating the skills with worked out examples; and following this by allowing the students to practise making the decisions in realistic situations such as case studies, role-plays and field exercises. More time and effort is required to learn those complex skills at the end of the

above list than the simpler ones given earlier. For example: knowledge about vitamins and food tables is required in order to practise the more advanced skill of calculating the vitamin content of a meal; knowledge about the advantages and disadvantages of different sources of water is required to practise the more complex skill of choosing an appropriate water source for a community.

Communication skills

Communication involves a combination of *decision-making skills* and *communication skills* including:

- choosing objectives;
- deciding actual content of advice, i.e. what to say;
- deciding which learning aids to use;
- ability to speak clearly and sufficiently loud to be heard;
- ability to listen, ask questions, promote discussion;
- use of non-verbal communication, including gestures, eye contact, tone of voice and posture, to establish rapport, show concern and encourage responses.

The best way of teaching communication skills is: first to demonstrate good communication to the learners; and then let everyone in the training group practise the skills with each other in role-plays. For example, you can ask someone to give a talk to the others who act as villagers and respond. Afterwards everyone can discuss how well the talk was done. You can give the audience a checklist like the one below to judge how well the communication was carried out.

- Was it interesting?
- Was it clear?
- Were the visual aids used well?
- Was there good use of questions?
- Was everyone encouraged to participate in discussion?

After everyone has had a chance to practise the communication skill, you can have a general discussion to bring out main points. You should encourage a friendly atmosphere of helpful criticism and explain that we can only learn by making mistakes and learning from them. However, if you feel that your students may be sensitive to criticism, you can give individual feedback afterwards. If a video camera is available it is a good idea to record the communication exercise so that they can see themselves afterwards. We all have mannerisms such as moving about, jangling keys, scratching noses, using favourite phrases and we often only realise it when we actually see ourselves! Once everyone has had a chance to try out the communication in a safe and friendly environment, you can let them try it out in a real situation with the community. This could involve asking them to teach a class with you observing and giving some feedback afterwards on how it went.

Psychomotor skills

Psychomotor skills involve learning how to perform manual operations such as threading film projectors, using drawing instruments, putting on a condom and giving injections. Often they are accompanied by decisions. For example, in addition to the skill of mixing oral rehydration solution, a mother would need to be able to decide how much and when to give the solution to her child. The decision-making and psychomotor skills can be taught separately.

Demonstration and providing opportunities to practise in pretend and real-life situations are the best ways of teaching psychomotor skills. For example, you could ask students to: put a condom onto a model of a penis; mix up oral rehydration solution and give it to a baby; add some oil to a weaning food and mix to the right consistency; build a latrine.

Attitudes

Attitudes involve a person's feelings towards something or someone. Attitudes are difficult to define and, because of this, are often left out of training programmes. However, it is not enough

to teach someone facts and skills. Whether the training is taken seriously and put into practice will usually depend on his or her attitudes. Some examples of important attitudes are:

- feeling that the topic of the training is important and should be put into practice;
- realising the importance of making follow-up visits;
- taking care and being accurate when measuring the weight of a child;
- being prepared to work among disadvantaged and poor people;
- being patient and prepared to listen to and respect the community;
- taking care to prepare one's health education properly.

Many people question whether it is actually possible to 'teach' attitudes such as commitment to working among poor people. They point to the importance of selection of people who already are motivated and show the necessary attitudes. However, there are several ways in which you can influence attitudes. One way is to provide opportunities for participants in your training programmes to discuss the importance of the attitudes involved.

Another way of developing attitudes is by personal example. Students often see their teachers as 'role models'. If you are trying to develop attitudes of sensitivity, commitment to work, thoroughness, accuracy, attention to detail, planning of work, one of the best ways of doing this is to set an example by your own personal behaviour. People will also be more likely to develop attitudes if they see that those attitudes are recognised and encouraged by their supervisors and employers.

In health education training we are often trying to develop respect and understanding of other people's point of view – empathy. A powerful method for developing empathy is to ask people to act out a situation in the community in a role-play, e.g. a woman receiving inappropriate health education on child feeding. Through role-play, a person can experience what it is like to be another person. Role-play is discussed in more detail later in this chapter.

Identifying types of learning

More examples of different kinds of learning applied to two very different topics – HIV/AIDS and eye health – are given in Table 4.1. You can practise recognising different kinds of learning with the example below. Look at the different activities in the list and identify types of learning separating them into simple knowledge, skills (thinking, communication and psychomotor) and attitudes. Check your answers against the correct ones. Once you are confident that you can distinguish different kinds of learning you can apply the checklist provided to help you plan your teaching.

Exercise on recognising different kinds of learning

1. Nurse knowing how to make a flip chart.
2. Village health worker being able to list the advantages of breastfeeding.
3. The ability to demonstrate to mothers how to give oral rehydration solution (ORS).
4. Clinic nurses wanting to spend time promoting latrines.
5. Nurses taking blood pressure.
6. Village health worker being able to list the sources of vitamin A.
7. Nurse choosing a balanced diet from available foods.
8. Nurse knowing the procedures for referral of TB patients.
9. Nurse deciding when to refer a patient to hospital.
10. Nurse being able to write down the different stages of the life cycle of the malaria parasite.
11. Nurse being able to plan how to prevent malaria in her community.
12. Nurse wanting to spend time in the community promoting malaria spraying.
13. Health assistant being aware of the services provided by the health education department.
14. Health assistant being aware of the importance of doing health education.

Answers: (1) decision-making (content of flip chart) as well as psychomotor (how to draw, bind pages); (2) factual knowledge; (3) factual knowledge about ORS, psychomotor skills in preparation of ORS,

communication skills; (4) attitude; (5) psychomotor skills and well as decision-making (6) factual knowledge; (7) factual knowledge of nutrients and sources of foods, decision-making as to choosing combinations; (8) factual knowledge of procedures (9) knowledge of procedures as well as decision-making skill of deciding in a given case whether to refer; (10) factual learning; (11) decision-making skill; (12) attitude; (13) factual knowledge; (14) attitude.

A checklist for analysing the learning components of your programme

- What information should the audience know by the end of the session?
  Either: simple facts *or* more complicated facts?
- What problem-solving or decision-making skills will they need to acquire?
- What communication skills do they need to acquire?
- What manual (psychomotor) skills should they be able to have by the end of the session?
- What attitudes should they have by the end of the session?

Setting objectives

Learning objectives are statements of the learning to be achieved by the end of the teaching session. They form the basis for planning of the content of the learning activities and for evaluation of the outcome. Learning objectives should specify:

- The exact learning required; *WHAT* is to change and by *HOW MUCH*.
- How the change will be measured, i.e. test conditions.
- The time over which the learning should take place.

The activities in a job description can form the overall objectives for a training programme. However, it is also helpful to set objectives for each type of learning needed to perform an activity.

An objective should be measurable. Psychomotor skills such as handling objects or communication skills (see below) are not difficult to measure as they can be directly

Table 4.1　Examples of types of learning for HIV/AIDS and Eye health programmes

Type of learning	Examples: AIDS and STDs	Examples: Eye health	Teaching method
Facts May be simple; or complex, familiar or new, compatible or in conflict with existing knowledge	The nature of AIDS and HIV; how HIV is and is not transmitted; how it affects the body; the effect of HIV on the body's immune system	The distribution, seriousness, cause and prevention of different blinding conditions; the role of flies in transmission of trachoma and onchocerciasis; the different kinds of refractive errors and how lenses can help	Teaching facts involves the following steps: relating the information to previous knowledge; presenting the information logically in a step-by-step fashion; using visual aids to explain relationships and avoiding presenting too much information in one session and causing overload.
Decision-making skills Involve application of knowledge to make decisions covering personal and family; life or one's professional role	Which mode of safer sex is most suited to one's lifestyle; how to select the best advice to meet a client's needs during counselling; how to set up an AIDS education programme in a workplace or community	How to promote eye health in one's own family; when to consult a doctor; how to control flies in the community; how to plan an eye health promotion programme in a workplace, school or community.	Decision-making skills are taught by: first providing the necessary basic information; then demonstrating the skills with worked out examples presented as case studies; then allowing the students to practise making the decisions in realistic situations such as case studies, role-plays and field exercises
Communication skills Verbal and non-verbal skills involved with giving information, persuading, and teaching	Negotiating with partner about safe sex and use of condoms; counselling a client on sensitive issues; giving a talk on AIDS; leading a group discussion	Explaining key eye health actions to family and friends; communicating effectively to patients; asking about feelings and needs and giving advice on preventive actions; giving a talk on eye health; leading a group discussion; using visual aids, etc.	First demonstrate good communication to the learners; and then let all trainees practise the skills with each other in role-plays. For example, you can ask someone to give a talk to the others, who act as the audience, or ask someone to give a counselling session. Afterwards, everyone can discuss how well the talk was done. It is helpful to video the session and let the person watch him/herself afterwards
Practical/manual skills **(Psychomotor skills)** Manipulating and handling objects	Putting on a condom correctly, disposing of injection needles safely; operating steam steriliser; disposal of infected materials	Examining the eye; washing the face; cleaning spectacles; making visual aids; building a pit latrine	Demonstrate the skill and provide opportunities to practise in pretend and real life situations

Table 4.1 Examples of types of learning for HIV/AIDS and Eye health programmes   *continued*

Type of learning	Examples: AIDS and STDs	Examples: Eye health	Teaching method
Attitudes and values *Feelings*	Confronting prejudice about homosexuals, sex workers and drug users and people living with AIDS/HIV; sensitivity, compassion, tolerance and patience in counselling; willingness to understand and respect other persons' viewpoints and maintain confidentiality	Realising the importance of prevention, increasing uptake of services, and bringing services to communities. The importance of gender sensitive approaches; respect for community values	Discuss the importance of particular attitudes; use role-plays where participants act out particular situations and experience what it is like to be another person, e.g. a woman receiving inappropriate advice, being blindfolded and having to move about. Involve persons affected by the problem in the training, e.g. blind, HIV positive. The trainers themselves should show consideration, concern, tolerance, commitment and provide a role model

observed. However changes in knowledge, thinking and attitudes are more difficult because they take place within a person's mind and not directly observable. We can only measure them by expressing them as actions – or *behavioural objectives*. This involves asking people to carry out actions such as to give opinions, describe situations, answer questions and undertake tests. Some examples of behavioural objectives are given here.

Some people are critical of using measurable objectives to plan and evaluate training activities. They feel that it can leave out changes in participants that are important but difficult to measure such as development of confidence, self-reliance and thinking skills – these are sometimes called personal growth. It also reinforces a 'top-down' approach which ignores the importance of the individual in deciding his or her own learning needs and outcomes. The critics of behavioural objectives would argue that the actual *process* of learning is as important as achieving particular outcomes.

However, a reply to this criticism is that if we cannot measure the purpose of the learning, the reason could be that we do not really know what we are trying to do! It would then be impossible to plan the programme or find out afterwards if we have been successful. In the past, training programmes have over-emphasised learning facts and we need to pay more attention to attitudes, decision-making

---

Examples of behavioural objectives

By the end of the session the participants:
- on being asked, will be able to list correctly the different stages of the life cycle of malaria (*knowledge*);
- on being taken to a house, will be able to choose the best location for locating a latrine (*decision-making*);
- in a test situation, will be able to use a flannelgraph to encourage learner participation in a small group teaching session (*communication skill*);
- on being given a pencil, ruler and paper will be able to enlarge a picture using the 'squaring up' method (*psychomotor*); and
- on being given data and a growth chart, will take care to enter data correctly onto a growth chart and recognise what follow-up advice is needed for the mother (*attitude/decision-making*).

and problem-solving. Also, we must recognise that training activities should not only concentrate on acquiring specific skills, but also include broader outcomes such as personal growth and the development of self-reliance. Chapter 6 will take up this discussion further when it considers the problem of setting objectives for community participation programmes and Chapter 11 will also look at objectives for programme planning and evaluation.

Some guidelines for promoting learning

Once you have undertaken the task analysis and identified the different kinds of learning you wish to promote, you can begin to choose your teaching strategies. Much attention has been put by educational psychologists into examining ways in which people learn and a summary of some of the lessons learned is given here.

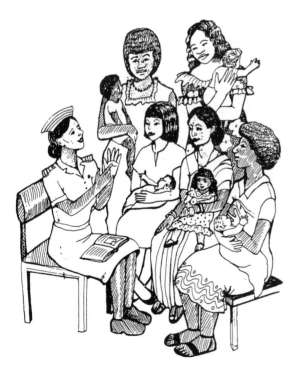

Fig. 4.3   We need to promote effective teaching and learning

Guidelines for effective teaching and learning

- People learn better if the information you present is linked to their experiences and builds on what they already know. Always ask questions at the beginning to find out what people know, think and feel about the topic.
- Your audience will only pay attention to you if the content of your teaching is relevant to what they want to know about, is put across in an interesting way and uses a variety of teaching styles.
- Complicated information should be introduced step-by-step in a logical organised way. Learning can be helped by well-chosen visual aids. Essential information can be on a handout and the time saved used for discussion.
- Take care not to overload your students with too many new ideas in one session as there is a limit to the amount of information that can be absorbed at one sitting. Use a range of teaching approaches such as talks, discussion, exercises and active learning methods. Build in frequent breaks between sessions where people can relax and stretch their legs. Twenty minutes at a time are probably the most people can concentrate.
- Information presented in a teaching session is quickly forgotten. Some further input, either by the student's own reading or reminders by the teacher, is needed for the information to be retained in long-term memory.
- Your audience may have enjoyed themselves and express appreciation but may not have learnt anything! The only way in which you can find out whether learning has taken place is by obtaining some feedback – either asking questions or observing their performance to see if they have improved.
- You should provide opportunities for your students to practise their newly-acquired skills in a safe, friendly and tolerant environment where they can make mistakes and receive helpful criticism without feeling threatened.
- People learn better if they are allowed to discover principles for themselves and activities are built into the learning process. Use active methods as follows:
  more active methods include: practice in real situations with supervision, practice in class situation, e.g. role-play; and discussion

less active methods: observing a drama or demonstration, looking at pictures, written examples, paper and pencil exercises; individual reading

SUMMARY

Active learning: make students think and apply the knowledge through a task.

Be clear: use visual aids, speak clearly, use simple language.

Make it meaningful: explain in advance what you are going to teach explain all new words and ideas; relate what you teach to student's lives and work; give examples; summarise main points at end.

Encourage participation: stimulate discussion and involve the group in the learning.

Ensure mastery: check understanding and competence reached.

Give feedback: tell the learners what their progress is.

Participatory learning

A serious criticism of many health education programmes is that they rely too much on traditional formal teaching methods where the audience is passive and simply listens. More emphasis is now placed on *participatory learning methods* and *dialogue* such as small-group teaching, simulations, case studies, group exercises and role-play. Participatory learning methods have many advantages. The participants are active and not passive so they are more likely to remember what was introduced during the session. They draw from their own experience. They are allowed to discover principles for themselves and can develop problem-solving skills. Participatory learning methods are especially relevant for those who did not do well at school. Other advantages of using a participatory approach are:

- it makes people think for themselves and be less dependent on you;
- it gives people greater pride in what they can do for themselves;
- you can discover the beliefs and practices of people in the community;
- it creates a close feeling between you and your group;
- it shows your interest and respect for the opinions of the community; and
- it also makes health education more fun!

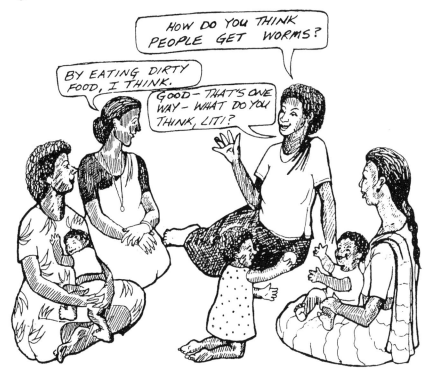

Fig. 4.4   Leading a discussion

One reason some people do not use participatory learning methods is shortage of time. A useful tip is to provide as much information as possible as handouts or a handbook. You can use the time saved for explaining difficult points, discussing important issues and introducing participatory learning methods.

Many people prefer giving a lecture and feel uncomfortable with the freer approach involved in a participatory learning situation. Sometimes they are worried that they will be asked questions that they can't answer. They can have problems getting a discussion going or dealing with individuals who dominate the class. If your audience is used to formal talks, they may feel shy about offering opinions and resistant to participatory methods. They may complain that you are not providing enough facts. Guidelines on leading a discussion are given below and more hints on working with groups are given in the next chapter.

---

10 tips for discussion leaders

1. Seating people in a circle is best for discussions. In a circle, there is no 'head' and everyone is equal. Sitting in a 'U' shape is the next best.
2. Tell your audience at the start that they will all be taking part in a discussion. Emphasise that you will NOT be doing all the talking.
3. Begin with easy questions. If you will be discussing more than one subject, begin with what you think people will be more free to talk about. This builds up people's confidence.
4. If you ask a question and no one answers, ask it again, using slightly different words.
5. Do not give up if answers are slow in coming. It will take people time to 'warm up' to this new way of learning.
6. Always respond with enthusiasm to any answer. Praise the people who answer, even if the answer is wrong: 'thank you for your thoughts', 'that's interesting'; and 'good for you for speaking up'.
7. Be sure to look around at everyone in the group. It is easy to look at only the one or two people who are answering all the questions and this discourages the others.
8. If someone asks you a question, a good way of keeping the discussion going is to direct the question back to the group: 'that's a very good question, Mrs Sharma, What do you think, Mrs Mthembu?'
9. The best discussions are short and leave people wishing for more. After an hour of so our minds begin to wander and not much more learning can take place.
10. Practice makes perfect! Before you lead the real discussion, it is very helpful to practise. Ask some of your family and friends to sit around and pretend that they are the people you will be speaking to. Ask them the same questions you will be asking your 'real audience', to find out what their response is.

Role-play

Role-play is the use of drama in which people act out situations for themselves in order to acquire communication and problem-solving skills and understand situations. Role-plays can vary in length between an extended session lasting a whole day to a 10-minute activity within a training class.

Role-play can help us learn more about ourselves and why we behave as we do. Role-plays can also help us to learn more about other people and their motivations. We can explore events from different points of view and develop empathy for communities. For example, men can act out the role of women and thus gain an understanding of the difficulties that they face in putting into practice health education messages.

Role-play is a very direct way of learning; you are given a role and have to think and speak immediately without detailed planning. Learning takes place through active experience; it is not passive. Role-play can be used to explore events that have already happened or which might happen. It uses situations that the members of the group are likely to find themselves in later in their lives. It gives group members the chance to consider different ways of responding within those situations. Some people find it easier to explain an experience through acting it out rather than reporting it or writing it down. Some examples of role-play activities are given below.

In role-play students can practise giving advice and making difficult decisions in a realistic situation. However, it is a 'safe' environment. You can make mistakes and try again which is not possible in real life, where mistakes could have disastrous consequences. It is possible to try several versions of the answer and the group can discuss which role-play it thinks best and why.

Examples of role-play activities used in training.

Ask a person to get into a wheelchair and move around a building to develop an understanding of what it feels like to be disabled.

Assign one person the role of a fieldworker and let the rest take on the roles of different members of a community. Have the fieldworker try to persuade the community to adopt a health practice, e.g. building latrines. After 10 or 15 minutes stop the role-play and have a discussion about how successful (or unsuccessful!) the fieldworker was and how his approach could be improved. Invite someone else to be the fieldworker and try a different approach.

Ask the group to take up roles of different members of a district health committee. One person acts as the health educator and tries to convince the others to work together to support a health education programme in the community. Problems of implementing health education programmes and overcoming bureaucratic resistance can be explored in the discussion afterwards.

Ask two people to act out a counselling situation with the others watching and afterwards discuss how successful it was. Another way of starting this is to use *role cards* (Figure 4.5) where situations are written down and a person has to pick one and the other has to respond. In the discussion afterwards people can list the good points of communication and the bad points and thus find out for themselves the principles of successful face-to-face communication.

Role-plays can help a group:

- to get to know one another better;
- to think about a particular topic, problem or issue;
- to practise for a particular event such as a meeting or interview;
- to be more sympathetic to points of view of other people;
- to acquire social skills such as cooperation;
- to acquire communication or counselling skills.

---

woman

You want us to build a latrine. If we do that it will mean more work cleaning and fetching water and I do not have enough time even now for my duties.

The fieldworker has to give advice to the person showing the card and thus learns to understand how a woman feels when faced with additional demands from hygiene education programmes.

Fig. 4.5   Example of a role card

Problem-solving exercises, case studies and simulations

The best way to develop problem-solving skills is to provide exercises where participants have to analyse a situation and decide on possible solutions. The problem can be in a real community or local clinic that the participants can visit and observe. You can then set a task which could be to:

- Design a leaflet on diarrhoea for mothers of under-fives.
- Suggest ways in which the health centre could improve its health education.
- Identify obstacles to promoting condoms; suggest how they can be overcome.
- Suggest how schools and primary health services could work better together.
- Make a work-plan for reaching out-of-school children and prepare an action plan.

Field visits can take up a lot of time and transport may not be available. It is often more convenient to use *case studies* in which the problem is presented to the students in the form of a written report describing a situation. Case studies can be long or short, complex or simple, depending on the needs of the participants, the nature of the subject matter and the time available. The case study can be designed to reveal problems such as the failure of a health education programme. You can base it on fact or a pretend situation, but it should be as realistic as possible. Enough background information should be included, as well as questions setting out the tasks for the participants.

Participants can work on the problem in groups of 4–8 persons. You can allow as little as one hour or, with more complex problems, half a day or more. Groups can present their conclusions to the other participants verbally or as a written report.

Case studies can be combined with other methods. For example, you might use the case study as the basis for a role-play. *Simulations* are case studies where the participants each take on particular roles. For example you might assign each member of a group the role of a person in a district health team so they tackle the problem 'in role'.

Games

You can present information and ideas on health in exciting and challenging ways through games. Games are entertaining, they encourage cooperation and discussion and they are good 'ice-breakers' at the beginning of a workshop to introduce participants and encourage an open approach to discussion. Some examples of games used in teaching about health include:

'Snakes and Ladders' where the snakes represent the causes of diarrhoea and the ladders are actions to prevent it.
Card game, e.g. a set of cards each containing a different activity that the participants have to sort out into low, medium and high risk for transmission of HIV virus.
'Chinese whispers' – one person whispers a phrase to another who has to whisper it to the next person until it has passed through every-

one. The final version is usually quite different from the original and in the discussion points are made about the distortion of messages that can occur through person-to-person communication in a community.

There are no fixed rules about how to go about developing a game. Start by deciding what knowledge and skills you want participants to learn. Use your imagination to think of interesting and different ways of communicating the points. Are there local games in your community that could be adapted?

Using learning aids to improve your teaching

Learning aids can greatly improve your teaching – but only if they are well-chosen and properly used. A learning aid is only an *aid* to learning. Just showing a film, picture or slide by itself will only have a limited effect. Rather than using

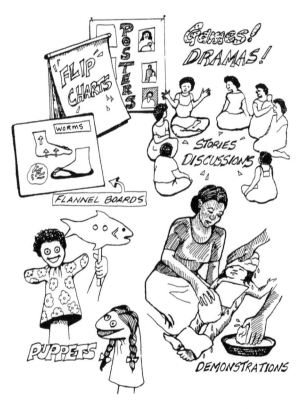

Fig. 4.6   Learning aids for teaching about health

them just for formal one-way teaching they should be used to stimulate understanding, discussion and participatory learning.

Learning aids can:

- keep the group's interest, arouse curiosity and hold attention;
- emphasise key points – when key headings are written out;
- allow step-by step explanation and sequencing of information;
- show something rather than just telling people – e.g. a jar of mosquito larvae, samples of condoms, drawing of a life cycle of a disease;
- provide a shared experience for discussion and questions.

An appropriate learning aid is:

- relevant to the learning objectives;
- affordable;
- easy to make and use;
- well understood by the audience;
- interesting and entertaining.
- It also encourages participation and discussion

Demonstrations with real objects and models

In Chapter 2 you saw how people were more likely to believe something if they can see, feel, touch and smell it for themselves. It is always best to use real objects as learning aids. You could set up a display of food, make a field visit to inspect a latrine, pass out condoms for people to inspect and blow into balloons to show how strong they are. However, it is often more convenient to use models rather than real objects. For example, models can be used to show a fruit which is out of season, a doll can be used to practise weighing or show the position of a baby during birth.

Using pictures in health education

Pictures can be useful learning aids if well chosen and properly used. Many kinds of *visual aids* use pictures.

- A picture put up on a wall is called a *wallchart*. Because the teacher is there to explain, wallcharts can contain more in-

formation than a poster that has to be understood on its own.
- A *flashcard* is a picture shown to a group of people; it can be a single picture but more often a series of pictures.
- It is easy to drop a set of flash cards by accident and mix them up. A *flip chart* is a series of pictures that are attached together – usually with a binding so they can be turned over one at a time.
- Other ways of using pictures include *flannelgraphs*, *slides* and *overhead projector transparencies*.

In the previous chapter you saw how easy it can be for people to misunderstand pictures. Wherever possible try to use the real thing or models – do not show a picture of a condom when you can show a real one. If it is not possible to show the real thing, a model might be easier to understand than a picture. If you decide to use pictures, pre-test them with a sample of your intended audience and make certain that they can be understood.

How pictures can be used to promote learning

Well chosen and properly used pictures can:

1. Convey visual information, e.g. what a latrine looks like.
2. Show something people cannot see in real life, e.g. internal structure of genital organs.
3. Provide a substitute for the real thing if difficult to obtain, e.g. pictures of out-of-season foods, a picture of child with particular symptoms.
4. Make difficult ideas easier to understand (*showing rather than telling*), e.g. making something small look larger, comparisons of similarities and differences, showing how something changes or grows, showing steps in doing a task.
5. Help people remember key points.
6. Arouse people's interest and gain attention.
7. Act as a stimulus for participatory learning and development of problem-solving skills, e.g. a picture posing a problem for which the group is invited to offer solutions, a sequence of pictures that the group is asked to put in an order that makes sense to them.

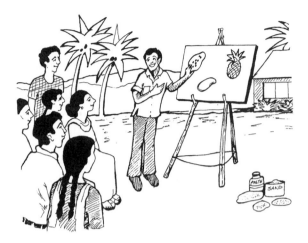

Fig. 4.7   The flannelgraph

Flannelgraphs

Flannelgraphs are pictures with a rough back which allows the picture to stick to a cloth. The picture can be printed on cloth or paper with a rough backing such as sandpaper. The board can be a blanket or cloth stuck to a board. Flannelgraphs have several advantages as visual aids:

- Flannelgraphs are easily carried by a field worker without a vehicle. They do not need electricity or expensive equipment to use.
- If they are properly stored, the pictures can be used repeatedly.
- They are simple and clear. They provide a visual framework on which to hang ideas.
- The subject can be built up picture by picture. Negative ideas can be replaced by positive ones and the scene can move and change.
- The pictures can be left up for as long as necessary for questions and discussion.
- They are quick to set up and use, in homes or in a group.
- They can be added to and adapted by the people using them.
- Flannelgraphs are easily used to encourage audience participation.

Slides

Slides or transparencies are photographs taken with 35 mm colour 'reversal' film that can be projected on a screen or white wall. Slides can be used to project colour photographs to a large size so a group of 20 or more people can see them. The organisation Teaching aids At Low Cost makes available slide sets on a wide range of health topics (see Appendix).

Slides can be used in many ways. You can encourage learner participation by inviting your audience to discuss what they see in the slide. Even better you can ask them to come forward and point out key topics.

You do not have to use all the slides in a set but can select the ones that are relevant to your need. This is especially useful if the slides have been produced in another country. Any 35mm camera can be used to take slides. So it is easy to take photographs locally either to make up a complete set or to include in one that you have bought.

Films and videos

Both films and videos have the advantage over 'still' photographs of showing movement and actions. This is particularly useful if you want to show skills such as building of a latrine or organising a drama session. They are also very good for attracting an audience and keeping their attention. However, one problem with films is that they need a blackout. Video does not need a darkened room, but the size of the screen is too small to use with a large group. Video projectors are available that can project onto a screen for larger audiences. If your audience is not familiar with film or video, there is a danger that they may see them as sources of entertainment rather than for instruction and learning. Never rely entirely on the film or video to convey the message. Always introduce the film beforehand to point out any special feature to look for and afterwards summarise and discuss with the group the key points to make sure that they have been understood. Some suggestions for using films and videos are given in the list.

Video programmes are easier to produce than film and you could try to find out if there are production facilities near you. You could even try to work with film makers to produce your own! Sometimes useful programmes are broadcast on the television and you can get permission to videotape them for use in your educational work.

The overhead projector

The overhead projector is a popular learning aid. It provides a bright picture in daylight so does not need a darkened room. When using it, you face the audience and do not have to turn your back to them. It is cheap to buy, simple to use and maintain. You can prepare transparencies in advance and when you finish your teaching, they can be stored for the next time you need them. Unfortunately many people do not use the overhead project to its best advantage and the words are too small, crowded and not clear. The guidelines in the list describe a range of imaginative and active ways of using the overhead projector and designing effective transparencies.

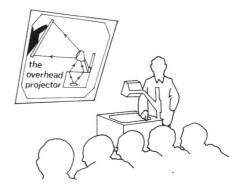

Fig.4.8   Using an overhead projector

Using films and videos

Questions to ask when choosing the film or video
1. Is the technical quality good – i.e. sound and picture quality?
2. What audience is it suitable for – children, the general public, health workers, student health workers, others?
3. Is it interesting?
4. Is it culturally acceptable to your audience and unlikely to cause offence?
5. Is it relevant and appropriate to your problems and your ways of dealing with them?
6. Is the health content accurate?
7. Can it be used to stimulate discussion?

Before showing it
Go early and set everything up, check that all equipment is working and the film or video is not damaged. Give a short introduction to the audience:
- give them hints about what to look for;
- explain words which they may find difficult;
- warn them about any parts of the film or video that you feel are not correct, or might distract them from the teaching points of the film; and
- make sure everyone has a clear view of the screen.

During the showing
Stay near the projector or video recorder in case there are serious problems or to adjust, the sound, focus etc.

After it is finished
Discuss the film with the audience. This lets you see whether they have observed the teaching points and explain any confusions.

Hints on using the overhead projector

MAKING THE TRANSPARENCIES
1. DESIGN your transparencies carefully. Plan them before you write them out.
2. KEEP IT SIMPLE – present one main idea on each sheet.
   - Aim for not more than 10 lines of lettering per transparency and maximum of seven words a line.
   - Use different colours to emphasise points (but do not use too many).
3. Always check that the words can be read from the back of the room. If you do copy diagrams make sure that they are large enough as most diagrams and words in books are too small. You might be able to obtain access to a photocopier which can enlarge pictures. Typewriting is too small, lettering should be at least 6 mm. Use lower case letters wherever possible as they are easier to read.
4. Try whenever possible to replace words with pictures. If you are not very good at drawing look out for pictures in books. It is easy to place a transparency over them to copy

5. Use a piece of lined paper under the acetate to keep your writing straight.
6. Margin – the edge of an overhead transparency is often not projected so leave 2 cm round the edge. It is a good idea to draw a border around the transparency as it focuses attention on the content.
7. Use overhead projector pens. Pens with water-based ink have the advantage of being easily erased with a damp cloth and the transparency can be reused. However, in hot humid conditions they easily smudge. 'Permanent' pens have a spirit-based ink. You can erase them within the first few minutes of use with methylated spirits but once they have dried they are difficult to remove and the transparency cannot be reused.
8. Acetate sheets for overhead transparencies come in different thicknesses – thicker ones last longer but are more expensive. Many photocopiers can copy diagrams onto special acetate sheets – check the instructions!

SHOWING THE TRANSPARENCIES

1. Position yourself, the projector and screen carefully – make sure the audience's view of the screen isn't blocked – and face the audience.
2. Switch off between transparencies – switching on the OHP is a signal and brings people's attention back to the screen.
3. Leave each transparency up long enough for the audience to absorb the information. Avoid the temptation to rush to the next visual.
4. Point out details on the transparency itself not on the screen. You can use a pen as a pointer.
5. Some of the different ways of using an overhead transparency include:
   - *transparency rolls* – writing points down as you go on rolls of acetate.
   - *'reveal method'* – covering the transparency with a sheet of paper that is lowered, step-by-step to reveal the words or pictures as you talk about them.
   - *masking* – masking off areas and revealing them in turn as appropriate.
   - *overlays* – one transparency laid over another to build up information and more detail.

Case studies of the use of different educational methods in health promotion

Health education among rural women in Bangladesh. A health education course was provided to five groups of 15 women – one topic per week over 12 weeks. The methods used involved demonstrations, practice and feedback supported by visual aids and handouts with pictures. At the end of the 12 weeks participants had retained 97% of the knowledge and just over half the women reported passing information to two relatives or neighbours.

Zigzaids game to teach young people about HIV/AIDS in Brazil. Zigzaids is a board game with 23 spaces that contain instructions for moving forwards or backwards. Players roll the dice to move along but must answer questions about AIDS contained in cards. Additionally, the game also includes 'surprise topics' that deal with such issues as haemophilia, blood transfusion, and drug action. A player wins by arriving first to the end, and his or her prize is a condom – called Zigzaids. The game also contained a leaflet for parents and teachers. The game was used in a variety of settings including classrooms, parents' meetings, vocational courses, day-care centres, company education programmes, supervision sessions for health workers etc. A total of 100,000 copies of the game were distributed, feedback from schools and other institutions was very positive and an observational study on children playing the game found changes in children's ideas and attitudes concerning the disease.

Using a game to teach growth monitoring in Kwa Zulu, South Africa. The 'Growth Monitoring Teaching Aid' is an educational game played over 2–4 hours at child health clinics. A bucket was attached to a weighing scale and mothers added water to increase the weight. An evaluation found that a group of mothers using the game had a higher understanding of growth monitoring and growth charts compared with similar mothers who had not used the game.

Promotion of home-made oral rehydration solution (ORS) in Bangladesh. The Bangladesh Rural Advancement Committee (BRAC) had originally sent its health workers to individual households, and mothers were trained to make up salt–sugar solution through a one-to-one approach. This approach was compared with a simpler approach using small group demonstration. A follow-up evaluation carried out one year later showed that both methods resulted in a similar increased use of ORS for children with severe diarrhoea. Group instruction was able to achieve the same levels of use of ORS at half the cost.

Promotion of oral rehydration in women from three rural villages in Ropar District of Punjab State, North India. The women in one group received verbal instructions on how to make up oral rehydation solution (ORS). Women from the second group were given the same verbal instructions and also a demonstration. The contents of ORS produced by the women who had been given the demonstration was chemically analysed and found to be near ideal and significantly better than that of the women who had only received instructions.

A cascade training approach to increase uptake of anti-malarial medicines in Nicaragua. A training course was held for a group of trainers who then trained 73,000 volunteers to mobilise the population to take a three-dose chloroquine regime. Educational activities made extensive use of media including newspapers, TV and radio as well as meetings at schools with parents, in the workplace, murals/posters, street megaphones and hanging of cloth signs outside houses. A follow-up survey found that about 70% of the population received anti-malarials and the malaria incidence reduced for 4 months following the campaign.

Hygiene education in urban slum communities in Dhaka, Bangladesh. Over a period of a week trainers and community health volunteers carried out small group discussions with women and children, larger demonstrations to mixed audiences and community-wide planning and action meetings to both men and women. Games, stories and posters were used to support the education. After the intervention more mothers washed their hands before preparing food in the intervention areas and there was a reduction in diarrhoea in children under 6 years old compared with a comparison community receiving no hygiene education.

Putting it all together – planning a lesson

You should now be in a position to apply the ideas presented above to planning your teaching.

Guidelines for giving a talk

ADVANCE PREPARATION AND PLANNING

1. Prepare the talk finding out the needs and background knowledge of the target group and size of group.
2. Write out objectives of the topic you want to put over.
3. Decide how much is to be covered in one session and ask:
   - What sequence should the information be presented in to make it as logical as possible?
   - What questions can I ask to check that the information is understood?
   - If skills are to be taught, how can I demonstrate the skill to the group? What opportunities can be provided to practise the skills either in the class or a real-life setting?
   - How can you best share the ideas you want to put across?
     o By having a discussion, demonstration, telling a story, acting out a drama?
     o By showing some pictures, playing a game?
4. Write an outline of your main points. (Avoid writing out the whole lecture, otherwise you will just read it out and sound boring.)
5. Prepare and practise using the visual aids you think will help in getting the information across.
   - Can key points and ideas be shown in pictures?
   - What learning aids can I use to explain these facts more clearly?
   - Can I put the most important information on a handout?
6. Check all the equipment, e.g. overhead projector, slide projector, extension cords, spare bulbs, etc. that you need are available and in good working order and the room is set up before the participants arrive.

RUNNING THE TEACHING SESSION

- Introduce yourself and the topic – get everyone's attention.

- Give a summary of the main points you will cover.
- Present your facts and information showing relevant visual aids when appropriate.
- Speak loud and clear so everyone can hear.
- Make sure your language is suited to your audience.
- Try not to be distracting by too much moving around or mannerisms, e.g. jangling keys.
- Keep a constant watch on the reactions of the group to your teaching. Look out for signs of misunderstanding or boredom in the class. Actively encourage questions.
- Provide practical assignments or reading to follow on from the lecture. Handouts listing the main points are often useful. Evaluate the session by asking questions or setting a task.

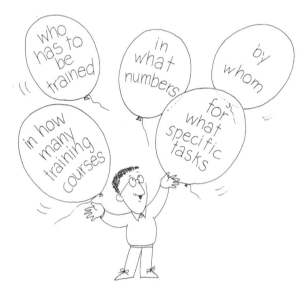

Fig. 4.9   Decision-making for planning training

Organising training programmes and workshops

Bringing people together is a costly process both in travel, food and disrupted work schedules. Face-to-face teaching sessions should be kept to a minimum. Concentrate on topics that *cannot* be learnt through distance learning such as attitudes, decision-making, communication and psychomotor skills. Can any of your objectives be achieved through distance learning methods?

These could be newsletters, talks on the radio or audio-cassettes and handbooks. The correspondence course is one form of distance education where reading materials, cassettes and even slides are sent to field workers with exercises and field activities. Feedback is given to the fieldworkers by post.

Once you have decided that a training workshop is needed you need to plan it properly. One of the biggest problems in training is ensuring that what has been learnt is actually applied in real life. Careful attention to the selection of participants, timing, place of training, content, teaching methods and follow-up will help to make sure that your training activities will be put into practice.

Selection of participants

You will have to consider carefully how you will make sure that you get the course participants you want. The ideal situation is to have participants who are of the right educational level and experience to benefit from the course, enthusiastic and motivated and can put into practice their newly-learnt ideas and skills. If you are running a community-based programme, the participants will probably have been chosen by the community themselves. It is important to get a good 'mix' of participants, especially male and female workers, background disciplines and experiences. Unfortunately, people may be sent for a training workshop for a variety of reasons – because of seniority, because it is their turn to have a 'day off' or personal connections.

Choice of place for training

Good teaching rooms, food and accommodation facilities are important; also, a training course will be more likely to be put into practice if it is carried out in a realistic field setting where relevant field exercises can be in the training.

Some people criticise the approach of bringing participants together to a training centre. An alternative is to run the training where people work so that all the fieldworkers in the local team can join in. This way they can discuss how they can put it into practice in their situation.

However, it is often a good idea to give people a chance to leave the pressures of their work to reflect on what they have been doing. A useful approach is to take two or three people from a single work setting. After the course they can continue to discuss what they have learnt and can support each other in putting the ideas into practice.

Timing the sessions

Carrying out all the teaching in one continuous course is not always the best approach. One way to encourage putting into practice is to split the training course into two or more blocks of teaching with gaps between. You can ask the participants to carry out reading and practical exercises in their workplace during the interval before their next course. When they come back together as a group you can then discuss the problems of putting the new ideas they have learnt into their practice. For example, if you have five days available for training you could use them in different ways as shown in Figure 4.10.

Organisation of the content

At the beginning of any training there should be a session to find out the background experiences of the participants and what they feel they need to know. This also helps to 'break the ice' and start the participants talking and getting to know each other. You can then introduce the aims of the training which you can change to take into account their interests. They are much more likely to pay attention and learn from their training if they have participated in discussions about the content and felt needs are met. You could even send out a questionnaire to all participants before the course begins to find out their views.

Keep the timetable flexible so that you can include any additional topics that arise and the participants want to discuss further. Include review sessions where you look back at what has been covered and look ahead at the next part of the programme. It is a good idea to ask the participants to select representatives who can bring to your attention any special needs and problems. Avoid the temptation to put in too much into a timetable. People need the opportunity to relax in the evenings and at meals otherwise they will get tired and lose concentration.

A good way of encouraging participants to put into practice their training is to provide a 'where do we go from here?' session at the end. They can prepare action plans for putting the new ideas into practice in their workplace and can present these plans to the other participants. You can follow this up with a discussion of possible obstacles to implementing their plans and how these obstacles can be overcome.

One problem with training courses is that they are taught as series of separate topics, e.g. how to do a community profile, advantages of community participation, use of educational methods. At the end of the course participants find it difficult to put it all into practice. An alternative to the traditional subject-based approach is a problem-solving approach to the teaching. This approach begins with a problem, e.g. how do we improve weaning practices in the community? How can latrines be promoted? How can we get young people to practise safe sex? Participants then carry out a series of activities in field situations to solve

'day release' one day per session	x	x	x	x	x
3-day course with two follow-up days	xxx		x		x
3-day course with 2-day follow-up course	xxx		xx		

x = one day's training

Fig. 4.10   Different ways of using five days for training

the problem. At various points in the course, trainers introduce key ideas. Participants will then be in a better position to apply the ideas gained in the course.

In one of my training courses at Leeds, I asked a group of students from Africa, Asia and the Caribbean to write down all the bad things they had experienced in workshops and all the good ones as well. The list of bad points was very long! Although workshops are widely used for introducing new ideas to fieldworkers, they are often not done very well. Typical problems are: overloaded and irrelevant content; poor facilities; inappropriate and overcrowded timetable; over-use of formal lectures and not enough discussion/practical activities; failure to consult the participants; poor organisation. It is not surprising that people do not put the ideas from workshops into practice! We followed up our discussions of good and bad points by preparing the 'Guidelines on running workshops' shown in the box on page 87.

Evaluation of training programmes

You will need to give some thought to how you will *evaluate* your workshop and some possible evaluation questions are listed here. Training programmes are evaluated for many different reasons: in the short term you will want to make sure that they have mastered the tasks and learning components in the course; in the long term you will need to find out if they are actually putting into practice the new ideas they have learnt and if they are having an impact on the health of the community.

Questions to ask when evaluating a training programme

Short-term evaluation

Were the participants satisfied with the content of the course?

Were there topics that they would have like to have seen included?

Was it taught in an interesting way?

Were the food, accommodation and social arrangements satisfactory?

At the end of the course were they able to perform to a satisfactory level the skills identified in the task analysis and course objective?

Do the participants feel confident that they can put into practice their new skills?

Is there a need for follow-up training?

Are there any general recommendations on policy from the participants?

Long-term evaluation

Are the participants satisfied with their training?

Do they have any further suggestions on training content?

Are the participants putting into practice what they have learnt?

What obstacles, if any, are preventing them from undertaking the newly-learnt skills?

Are their employers satisfied with the results of the training?

Is the community satisfied with the results of the training?

What impact have their activities had upon the health of the community?

Is there a need for follow-up training?

Summary

This chapter has looked at some of the issues you should consider in planning effective programmes of teaching and training. The main points can be summarised as:

1 Decide on the overall objectives for the teaching; this is done by analysis of the tasks to be performed and involvement of the participants themselves.

2 Analyse the kinds of learning involved in carrying out the tasks; this involves identifying the need for learning facts, skills (decision-making, psychomotor and communication) and attitudes.

3 Choose appropriate teaching methods for each type of learning; include active methods of learning including problem-solving, role-play and field exercises; select appropriate learning aids.

Guidelines on running workshops

Before the workshop
- Form an organising committee to plan the workshop with clearly-defined responsibilities for each member.
- Have clearly-defined objectives for the workshop; specify date and length of the workshop.
- Decide who the participants will be and how many should come; visit participants and their managers where possible in their workplace to discuss the workshop and ask for suggestions on content. Where a personal visit is not possible, send a questionnaire to participants in which they can identify their needs; send out invitations to participants well in advance; check that they can come and have a reserve list if people drop out.
- Identify external speakers and chairpersons for sessions; have meetings with resource persons and facilitators to brief them and identify any required resources; identify a person to open and close the workshop; give everybody plenty of notice; check they can come.
- Choose the place where the workshop is taking place including the accommodation, teaching rooms; locations for field visits; inspect and check lighting, size, seating, recreational facilities during evening, toilet facilities; speak to the local administrator of the facility (and the catering officer if a separate person) and explain requirements; confirm the booking.
- Plan the timetable; prepare a social programme with some visits and evening activities.
- Arrange for typing and duplicating facilities during the workshop.
- Make a budget providing for transport, hire of rooms, food, accommodation, materials, speaker's expenses, hire of equipment, secretarial expenses; submit to finance office and ensure approval and that money is available.
- Order required materials, stationery, pens, paper; arrange for printing of handouts and timetable; obtain any learning aids required including flip charts, videos etc.
- Invite media to opening and close of the workshop and send out a press release.

During the workshop
- Register participants; issue name badges, timetables, notepads; organise financial arrangements.
- Brief participants (introduction and 'icebreaking').
- Give out a pre-test questionnaire to participants (if one had not been given before); discuss the participants' expectations.
- Form a workshop committee with involvement of participants.
- Make yourself available to sort out problems as and when they occur.
- Obtain feedback at end of each day; get proceedings of each day typed up; monitoring timetable where necessary.
- Keep a written record of any recommendations and resolutions.
- Evaluate at end of the workshop.

After the workshop is over
- Return all borrowed equipment and materials.
- Prepare report with the workshop recommendations and send it to decision-makers, sponsors and participants.
- Write to all resource persons and thank for participation.
- Pay all outstanding bills and produce final budget.
- Hold meeting of organising committee to discuss workshop report and follow-up.

---

4   Prepare a plan for the training; decide on selection of participants, duration and timing of training, location of training, timetable for the programme, resources (equipment and staff), and assessment of performance.

5   Carry out short-term and long-term evaluation of the teaching activity.

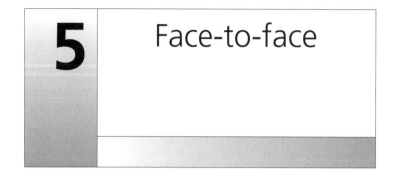

5 Face-to-face

This chapter will look at some of the ways in which you can work effectively with individuals and small groups. It will build on the discussions of communication and teaching methods in the previous two chapters and explore:

1 different kinds of *one-to-one* communication ranging from simple instruction to problem-solving counselling and how these can be carried out;
2 the role of groups in health education and health promotion and methods for working in groups;
3 ways in which the effectiveness of face-to-face communication can be improved;
4 putting face-to-face communication into practice in patient education programmes.

In previous chapters many advantages of face-to-face or 'person-to-person' communication were discussed. Face-to-face methods have a number of advantages over mass media such as radio or leaflets. It is possible to make the advice specific to the needs of your audience. You can find out how much they know already by asking questions at the beginning of a session and change the advice you are giving. You can also ask questions at the end of a session and discover how well understood and convincing you have been!

Non-verbal communication

Face-to-face communication involves many different kinds of communication. The most obvious communication takes place through the actual words – *verbal communication*. You will already have looked at communication difficulties from using complicated unfamiliar words in Chapter 3. Unfortunately some people deliberately use long technical words as a means of showing off and acting in a superior way.

Much communication also takes place through *non-verbal communication* which was also introduced in Chapter 3. Table 5.1 summarises the many different kinds of non-verbal communication that includes all those aspects of communication between people that do not involve the actual meaning of words. Most of us think a great deal about choosing the words we say when talking with another person. However, we often forget to plan our non-verbal communication. But the gestures we use, how we look at people, our tone of voice, how we are seated and our clothes can all have an impact on the way people interpret what we say.

We use non-verbal communication continually in every-day contact. For example, you might decide that a person is not telling the truth because he doesn't 'look' convincing. People express anger, love, sympathy and other emotions through their non-verbal communication. Points in conversations are emphasised through gestures and head nodding. An important feedback on whether people are listening comes from nods, sounds of agreements 'ums and ahs' and looks of encouragement (see Table 5.1). It is a useful exercise just to watch people

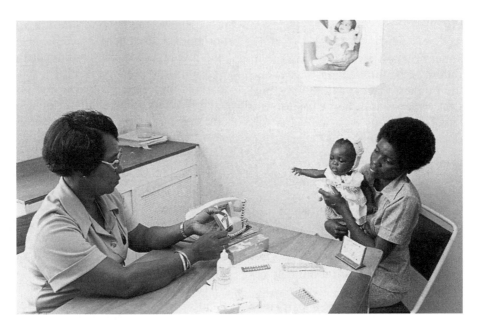

Fig. 5.1   Face-to-face communication has many advantages

talking and look out for non-verbal communication. You can also learn a great deal about non-verbal communication by turning down the sound when watching television or speeding up the motion on a video recorder.

In your face-to-face communication you have to be sensitive to the impact your non-verbal communication might be having. For example: sitting behind a desk can reinforce the barrier between health worker and community; looking at your watch, looking away or writing down notes might be taken as showing boredom; and talking loudly may seem a sign of anger.

Non-verbal communication can be interpreted in different ways according to the culture of the community and this can also lead to misunderstandings. For example in western cultures much importance is given to looking people straight in the eye. In other cultures looking directly at someone in the face can be considered rude and showing lack of respect. Greetings and ways of showing sympathy can vary according to the culture.

So in your contacts with other people, either individually or in groups, you have to become sensitive to your own non-verbal communication. It is not enough listening, feeling sympathetic and concerned for the other persons. You have to be able to *show* it.

Table 5.1   Different kinds of non-verbal communication

Sounds accompanying spoken words
pitch of voice
'um's, er's' and other sounds
laughing, angry, groaning
pauses
speed of talking
stresses on particular words
loudness or softness

Body language

body contact	touching, holding hands, caressing greetings, shaking hands
closeness	distance between persons
posture	sitting up, slouching, leaning forward
orientation	angle at which people put themselves
gestures	hand movements, shaking and nodding head
gaze/looks	eye movements, raising eye brows, shape of mouth
appearance	clothes, hair, cleanliness

One-to-one

The one-to-one situation is very important in health education. Situations where one-to-one communication takes place include meetings between doctors and patients, home visits in the community and discussions with individuals in communities and can include:

- simple giving of information;
- persuading someone to undertake a particular action;
- helping someone to take a decision, e.g. which contraceptive method to use;
- breaking sensitive news, e.g. that the person is infected with HIV virus;
- helping someone to cope with a difficult situation; and
- therapy for someone who has a particular problem, e.g. is an alcoholic.

Counselling

In traditional advice giving, the health worker is often trying to persuade a person to follow a particular course of action. Counselling is a process that goes beyond simply giving information but involves helping people *to make decisions* and giving them the confidence to put their decisions into practice. A difficulty we all have is to avoid imposing our own views on others. We need to try to understand our own values, opinions and prejudices so that we don't impose our own values on others. Counselling is based on the following assumptions:

- Counselling should take into account psychosocial, financial and spiritual needs of the client.
- Everything said during a counselling session should be treated as strictly confidential.
- Any information provided should be clearly put, accurate and consistent.
- The emphasis should be that of promoting informed decision-making; the counsellor avoids giving direct advice but instead helps the person to make decisions for themselves.
- The client has the right to choose his or own actions.

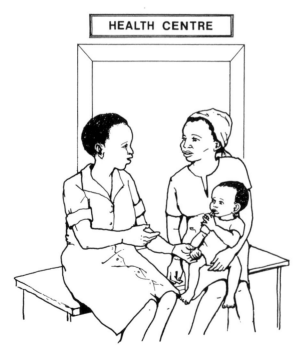

Fig. 5.2 One-to-one communication

Eight common reasons for breakdown of one-to-one communication

1. The communication is carried out in a place where there is a lot of noise and distractions.
2. The person feels uncomfortable and distracted, is too self-conscious to discuss problems because of people overhearing or does not really trust health educator.
3. The health educator doesn't find out the real reasons for the problem, uses complicated language with unfamiliar terms, and gives advice that is irrelevant or impossible to put into practice.
4. People go away with doubts and questions that they felt that they could not raise with the health worker.
5. Most people want to be told more about their illnesses than the doctor is willing to say.
6. Too much information is given; the person only remembers part of what was said during the meeting – especially if he/she is anxious and worried during the consultation.
7. There is a wide difference in background between the two persons without enough

sharing of culture, perceptions, beliefs and values to allow communication and understanding. Insufficient time is available to find out what the person's problems really are or properly explain the facts.

8. There is no follow-up to check if the advice is put into practice.

Promoting effective one-to-one communication

Many studies have been carried out on communication between health workers and their patients to find out the reasons why patients do not follow the advice given. Some of the problems that these studies have identified are shown in the list and Figure 5.3.

For effective one-to-one communication three sets of factors are important to consider: the place and time when the communication takes place; the handling of the actual encounter; and obtaining feedback on the effectiveness.

The place and time

If you are seeing people at a health centre, you should try to set aside a place where you can talk to them in private without interruptions. If you do not have much time to spare, or have others to see as well, you can ask the person to return later when you have more free time. If you have a receptionist to answer the telephone, ask for any calls to be intercepted during the session.

Handling the encounter

The way you conduct your session – talking and listening – will have an impact on its effectiveness. You may find the GATHER approach described on p. 92 a useful check list as well as the guidelines below:

- Put the person at ease at the beginning of the session with a smile and a greeting.
- Choose carefully what advice to give so that it is relevant, and realistic; be selective about the amount of information you give in any one session. The more information you provide the more likely it will be that the person will forget what you are saying – try to aim to make three or four key points.
- Make your advice as specific as possible – instead of saying 'practise good hygiene' say 'wash your hands before preparing your baby's food'.
- Use simple language – avoid technical terms.
- Give information in an organised way: 'I am going to tell you three things you can do. The first is........The second is .... and the third is......'
- Give the most important advice first and repeat it at the end.
- Check that your main points have been understood by asking questions such as 'now please explain back to me how often you should take the pills'.
- Provide a leaflet with the key points for the person to take away.

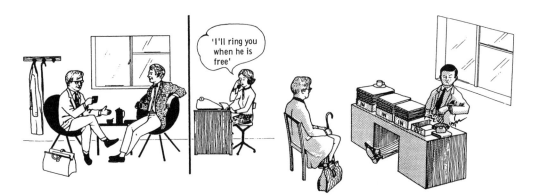

Fig. 5.3   Blocks to communication. What difference do you see between the two situations in the illustration?

We often are so concerned with giving advice that we do not listen to what people themselves want to know. *Listening* is an important part of handling the encounter. Some common problems in listening include the following:

- *daydreaming* – because we can think faster than people can talk to us we can easily become distracted and think of other things and miss important points;
- *jumping to conclusions* – we jump to conclusions about what people are going to say so we don't really pay attention;
- *reacting to specific words* – we react strongly to certain words such as money, lack of time, family problems and stop listening; and
- *turning off* when the subject is complicated – if the topic is complicated and involved we can turn off and stop listening.

When you are listening to someone, try to avoid: passing judgement either in words or through your looks and gestures; arguing; interrupting and rushing them and jumping to conclusions. Listening is an *active* process. You should continually show interest and provide encouragement and pay attention by looking at the person. Try to give the person time to explain their situation and don't be afraid to allow moments of silence while they are collecting their thoughts. You should ask or clarification on any points you don't understand.

Obtaining feedback on the outcome of the session

This is the third ingredient for effective one-to-one communication. This can be asking questions. For example you could ask what the person intends to do and whether he or she feels that they can put into practice the advice you have given. You will have to ask in a sensitive way; you might be told what they think you want to hear rather than what they really believe. You could ask the person to return at a future date when you can look for improvements in health. You could also make a follow-up visit to the person's home or ask someone else to pay a visit and observe their progress.

The GATHER approach to one-to-one communication

G *Greet the person*: put them at ease, show respect and trust; emphasise the confidential nature of the discussion.

A *Ask about their problem*: encourage them to bring out their anxieties, worries and needs, determine their access to support and help in their family and community; find out what steps they have already taken to deal with the situation; encourage the person to express their feelings in their own words; show respect and tolerance to what they say and do not pass judgement; actively listen and show that you are paying attention through your looking; encourage them through helpful questions.

T *Tell them any relevant information* they need: provide accurate and specific information in reply to their questions; give information on what they can do to help their health, explain any background information they need to know about the particular health issue; keep your language simple, repeat important points and ask questions to check that the important points are understood; provide the important information in the form of a leaflet that they can take away.

H *Help them to make decisions*: explore the various alternatives; raise issues they may not have thought of; be careful of letting your own views, values and prejudices influence the advice you give; ensure that it is their own decision and not one that you have imposed; help them make a plan of action.

E *Explain any misunderstandings*: ask questions to check understanding of important points; ask the person to repeat back in their own words the key points you have made.

R *Return to follow up on them*: make arrangements for a follow-up visit or referral to other agencies; if a follow-up visit is not necessary, give the name of someone who they can contact it they have need for help.

Working with groups

There are many different reasons why we work in groups for our health education and health promotion work.

Problem-solving groups and teams

Planning and implementing your educational activities will usually involve setting up groups such as committees or working in teams with other people. You may need to set up groups in order to: solve problems and make decisions, bring together a set of skills, talents and responsibilities to find the best possible solution to a problem; collect information and ideas; gather ideas, information or make suggestions; and co-ordinate the activities of different persons.

Teaching/learning groups

You will already have seen in the previous chapter that teaching with small groups has many advantages. You can use groups to: develop problem-solving skills; encourage learner participation, discussion and feedback; explore values and beliefs; and deal with sensitive issues such as sex.

Community-based groups

Community participation programmes usually set up committees to manage the programme, make decisions and liaise with the health services (see Chapter 6). The success or failure of community participation programmes will depend heavily on how well these groups function and how much support they receive from field-workers.

Self-help groups

Belonging to a small group can benefit members directly through the help they can give each other. Support and practical advice from someone else who has had a similar problem is often more useful than receiving advice from a health worker. Many people with problems can feel very isolated and find it helpful to meet others with similar experiences. Self-help groups have been set up on many different topics and some examples are given here.

The different kinds of groups described above overlap. You might set up a group within a community-based programme and then undertake some small group teaching activity with it. You

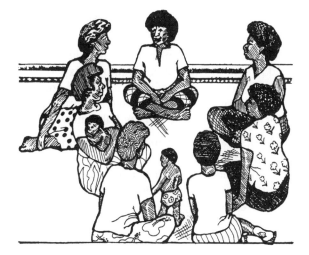

Fig. 5.4   Group discussion

Examples of self-help groups

Alcoholics Anonymous where all the members are alcoholics and help each other to stop drinking.
Breastfeeding support groups where women who are breastfeeding meet, share experiences, help each other and receive help from other women who have successfully breast fed.
AIDS Support Groups e.g. 'Body positive' – groups of persons who are HIV antibody positive regularly meet to provide each other support and encouragement.
Colostomy support groups – people who have had a colostomy operation involving removal of part of their colon so that their faeces emerge from an opening on their side into a plastic bag. This support group involves meeting and sharing experiences, discuss coping strategies, briefing people who are about to have the operation.
Stop smoking groups – people who want to give up smoking forming a group and regularly meet to provide support and monitor each other's progress.

may hold a group teaching session with patients at a clinic, e.g. leprosy patients and encourage them to continue as a self-help group to provide each other mutual support. You might form a liaison committee to run a health education programme in your district and conduct a small group teaching session to introduce a new skill.

Problems in group functioning

Working in groups can be highly effective and get good results. It can also be frustrating, difficult and lead to failure. Think about your own experiences with groups – what problems have you encountered? Have any of your own experiences of difficulties included any of the following?

• Lack of a common purpose; everyone wants something different.
• Some individuals dominate the discussion, others are silent and do not contribute.
• There are disagreements, personality clashes and conflicts among the members.
• Members fail to perform assigned tasks.
• Attendance is poor and irregular.
• Everyone talks but nobody is willing to make decisions.

Group dynamics

The functioning of groups has been called *group dynamics*. Social psychologists have studied group dynamics and have found the following to be important in determining the effectiveness of group functioning: the characteristics of the group including size and membership; the nature of the tasks undertaken; the decision-making processes; the roles of members; group processes; and pattern of leadership.

Characteristics of the group

Here are some definitions of what constitutes a group:

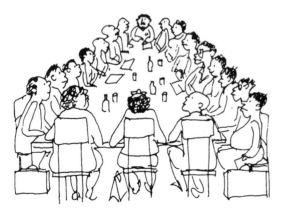

Fig. 5.5   Meetings

'...a group is best defined as a dynamic whole based on interdependence rather than similarity' (Lewin)
'... the distinctive thing about a group is that its members share norms about something' (Newcomb)
'... engaged in interaction with one another in a single face-to-face meeting or series of such meetings' (Bales)

A group is not just a collection of people – they should *share some characteristics and interact*. Because of this interaction, a group is more than the sum of the individuals that make it up. The group acquires its own characteristics.

Size of group

A group can have as few as four people and as many as 24. The kinds of interactions, opportunities for exchange of ideas and success in achieving objectives are affected by the group size. With too few members most people will have a chance to contribute, but there will be less experience to draw on from the members. With too many people, it is difficult for everyone to contribute in discussion and it will be harder to reach a shared decision. Many feel that 8–12 persons is an ideal size for a group but it really depends on the aims and purpose of the group.

Background of the group members

Who the group members are and their reasons for attending are of enormous importance. If the members have been sent by their employers to attend, they may not really be interested in the group – they may even feel that their selection is a punishment. Persons may have a 'hidden agenda' and see the function of the group as meeting their own personal or employer's wishes. Other ways in which individual behaviours help or hinder the group are described below in the section on group processes. You may have no choice but to accept into the group whoever has been sent. However, wherever possible try to involve people who you know will work well with others.

The nature of the task

Some of the different kinds of tasks that groups are concerned with were described at the beginning of this section. Another way of thinking about different kinds of groups is the extent to which they are mainly concerned with producing results (task-oriented) or with promoting the well-being of the members of the groups (process-oriented) – see Figure 5.6.

Group decision-making

Every group is constantly making decisions. Some decisions may be small, others may be large ones with important consequences. How well those decisions are made will depend on many factors including: complexity of the decision required; the range of skills/expertise in the group and the amount of relevant information available to the members. One way of reaching a decision in a group is through *consensus* – with everyone's agreement. This is often the best way – provided you are sure that everyone really does agree and not just keeping their disagreement silent because they feel inhibited to give their opinion. With a larger group it can be difficult to get everyone to agree. A vote can be taken and the majority view followed. But if you do make decisions by voting, you must take care that those with minority views do not feel left out and drop out of future activities.

Some of the different reasons why groups find it difficult to make decisions are given here. To overcome these problems, the group must be honest with itself and openly discuss them and

try to find a solution. Good leadership is essential to resolve these difficulties and make effective decisions.

Individual roles of members

During a group's activities, members can take a range of roles – some helpful and others unhelpful. A workshop held in Zambia by the Economic Commission for Africa identified the following characteristics and provided hints on how to deal with them.

The quarrelsome type. Keep cool. Don't allow yourself to become involved in an argument. Ask them questions and they will probably make some foolish or far-fetched statements that can be dealt with by other group members. Don't allow anyone to become personal.

The positive type. They can be of great help to the chairperson, particularly when the discussion gets bogged down. Use them frequently but don't let them monopolise the conversation.

The know-all type. They may be bluffing and not really know the answers. When they give an opinion ask them to give reasons. If the reasons seem faulty ask other members of the group to comment. This helps to build up confidence in the group so they will not be imposed on.

The talkative type. Don't discourage them. If they are well-informed their opinion can be of help to

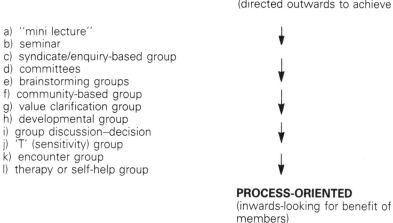

TASK-ORIENTED
(directed outwards to achieve tasks)

a) ''mini lecture''
b) seminar
c) syndicate/enquiry-based group
d) committees
e) brainstorming groups
f) community-based group
g) value clarification group
h) developmental group
i) group discussion–decision
j) 'T' (sensitivity) group
k) encounter group
l) therapy or self-help group

PROCESS-ORIENTED
(inwards-looking for benefit of members)

Fig. 5.6   Process and task-oriented groups

Obstacles to group decision-making

- **Fear of consequences**: fear that employers or other influential people will criticise them for taking a particular decision.
- **Conflicting loyalties**: there can be divided loyalties among the different members to employers, communities, churches etc.
- **Disagreements and personalities**: personal behaviour and disagreements between group members can interfere with decision-making (see section on individual behaviour).
- **Hidden agenda**: individual group members may try to influence the whole group to follow their particular interests.
- **Inadequate information**: the decision may be made based on the personal opinions of the group members rather than the facts of the situation.

the group. If they talk for too long they can bore others. Be prepared to interrupt them tactfully and ask a direct question of someone else.

The shy type. They may know a great deal but be shy to speak out. Often the talkative and know-all types are the men; the women may be more shy but have much of importance to contribute to the group. When suitable opportunities come, call upon them by name to give an opinion but be sure that the question is an easy one to build up confidence to contribute more to the group.

The uncooperative rejecting type. Be patient and try to win their friendship. Acknowledge his experience and let them feel that you depend upon their help for the success of the meeting.

The highbrow intellectual type. Be patient, but keep to the point; if necessary, rephrase their statements for the benefit of other members. Ask them to help the group with difficult technical points. Take care that they do not over-awe the rest of the group and make them feel inadequate.

The persistent questioner. They are often out to trap the chairperson. Pass their questions back to the group and then get the questioner's views.

Other types of difficult group behaviour were identified in that same workshop and given the personalities of animals!

The *donkey* – who is very stubborn and will not change his point of view 'I will not be moved'.

The *lion* – who fights whenever others disagree with his plans or interferes with his desires.

The *rabbit* – who runs away when he senses tension or conflict or switches quickly to another topic.

The *ostrich* – who buries his head in the sand and refuses to admit any problem at all.

The *monkey* – who fools around and prevents the group from concentrating on serious business.

The *hyena* – who laughs and makes jokes to avoid dealing with difficulties or puts rivals down.

The *elephant* – who blocks the way and stubbornly prevents the group from continuing along the road to their desired goals.

The *giraffe* – who looks down on others and on the programme in general feeling that 'I am above it all'.

The *tortoise* – who withdraws from the group, refusing to give ideas or opinions.

The *cat* – who is always looking for sympathy. 'It is so difficult for me'.

The *peacock* – who is always competing for attention. 'See what a fine fellow I am'.

Stages in setting up a group

One useful approach shown in Table 5.2 is to separate out the various stages of establishing a group into: the setting up stage or 'forming'; the action stage or 'storming'; and the establishing stage or 'norming'. Some of the issues you should consider at each stage are shown in Table 5.2 and you will probably notice some similarities with the stages in community participation described in Chapter 6.

In the setting up stage it is essential to create a climate of trust. Everyone should feel free to give their opinion, share ideas and be prepared to work together to achieve the objectives. You have to look out for people who have hidden reasons for attending. Others may have come only because they have been told to attend by their employers but are really not very interested. Have you left out anyone important from the membership?

Table 5.2 Stages in group formation and action

SETTING UP	create climate of trust between members share expectations understand each person's personal objectives agree on objectives for group review membership and involve others if needed agree on strategy for achieving objectives
ACTION	obtain necessary data set up working groups make decisions implement activities
ESTABLISHING	evaluate activities reflect on achievements review objectives make future plans review membership and involve others if necessary, decide to end group

The action stage depends a great deal on the quality of leadership, which is discussed below. Only a limited range of topics can be handled in detail by a group at any one meeting. Large meetings are good for obtaining agreement on broad points. However, they can be inefficient for detailed work such as preparing a curriculum, writing a leaflet etc. It is better to delegate these tasks to individuals or working groups. The products of these working groups can later be discussed at a full meeting.

The establishing stage can be time for expansion. However, it is also a time when a group can become fixed in its ways and inward-looking. The challenge at this stage is to find ways of maintaining the enthusiasm and energy of the members.

Leadership and effective group functioning

How well a group performs depends a great deal on the leadership. Studies of group dynamics point to a wide range of approaches to leadership. These fall along the spectrum shown in Figure 5.7 ranging from a *laissez-faire* ('leave it to the members') approach through to a top-down authoritarian ('I am in charge') approach.

The authoritarian approach can reduce creativity and ideas from the members and limit the output of the group. *Laissez-faire* can result in chaos and muddle. The best approach is one where the leader acts as *facilitator* and helps everyone to work together – but when necessary can provide some strong pressure on the group members as a stimulus to action if the meeting has become bogged down and is failing to reach a decision.

It is helpful to separate out the role of the group leader into two broad areas: *task maintenance functions* are those activities which help to get the group's task done:

setting the agenda
 'Today our priority is to plan next year's programme'
introducing new information
 'Funds are available for a leaflet'
asking for further information
 'How much will this cost?'
making things clear
 'I think what Jim means is …'
summarising present position
 'We are now agreed to set up a drama project'

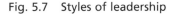

authoritarian		democratic		laissez-faire
leader orders group	leader persuades group	leader consults group	leader shares decisions with group	leader leaves decision-making to group

Fig. 5.7   Styles of leadership

inviting suggestions from members
'Does anyone have any suggestions for how we can …?'
prodding
'There's ten minutes left to make a decision on this'
trying to find new ways around a problem
'Let's think again how we can solve this'
reviewing objectives
'Let's remind ourselves that our main aim is to find a way of reaching men with our safe sex message'
introducing brainstorms, buzz groups (see below)
'Let's try a brainstorm to see if we can get some new ideas'

Group maintenance

Group maintenance functions of a leader are those dealing with the 'well-being' of the group. This might involve:

- dealing with difficult group members;
- encouraging quieter members to participate;
- dealing with conflicts;
- seeking consensus;
- lightening the tension; and
- expressing group feelings.

In Chapter 4 the value of participatory learning and group discussion was looked at in some detail. The 'Ten Tips for Discussion Leaders' presented on page 76 suggest how you can encourage group members to take part in discussions. Brainstorming and buzz groups are two more methods that can help improve the effectiveness of groups to make decisions and solve problems.

The *brainstorming* method is an approach for getting a large number of ideas from a group quickly. Suppose you were wishing to think of some possible ideas for a campaign to get the newspapers to publicise accidents in the home. In a typical discussion group, one person suggests an idea and the group discusses it. Then a second person suggests another idea and that is also discussed. At the end of the session you may only have discussed a few suggestions. The quieter persons may have some good ideas but have been too shy to say them aloud. In the brainstorming approach you get the group to generate a list of ideas – and discuss them afterwards.

Brainstorming:

- Place people in a circle and explain to them that you want their ideas and suggestions.
- Emphasise that they should use their imagination and be creative – but no-one should comment on each other's suggestions until later.
- Ask one person to write down each suggestion on a large sheet of paper.
- After 5 or 10 minutes you should have a long list of ideas. You can then pick out the ones that look the most useful.

If you want to find solutions to problems more quickly you could always try dividing them into smaller groups and giving a fixed time limit to produce some suggestions. You may not have enough time for discussion groups and one simple approach is to form *buzz groups*. Ask each member of the group to turn to their neighbour to make small groups of two or three persons. Ask them to discuss the points and give them a time limit of 5 minutes to produce some suggestions.

In addition to the suggestions on leadership roles and group discussion methods given above, some guidelines on running successful meetings are listed here.

Things to do to make meetings work

1. Prepare an agenda and circulate it with any background papers well in advance.
2. Check out the agenda in advance and make sure you are well prepared.
3. Arrange the seating – make sure it is in a circle.
4. Start the meeting on time.
5. Agree at the beginning on the finishing time – this focuses everybody on the task ahead.
6. Welcome any new members and invite them to introduce themselves.
7. Provide some refreshments if people have come from a long way or the meeting is more than an hour in length.
8. Chair the meeting to ensure order and participation by everyone.
9. Finish on time – if necessary, put off unfinished business to the next meeting.
10. Thank everyone for their contribution.

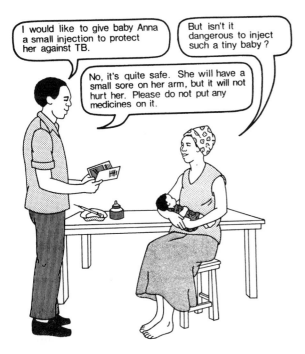

Fig. 5.8   Patient education

Patient education

According to WHO an average of only 50% of patients worldwide take their medicines correctly. Patient education is the name for one-to-one and group education provided to patients in clinics and hospitals as part of the treatment and rehabilitation process and covers adherence to treatment and other changes in lifestyle needed to support recovery of the patient. Typical examples of patient education would be:

- explaining how much, how often and when medicines should be taken and possible side effects;
- explaining why a medicine may not be needed in some situations (important to prevent the unnecessary use of antibiotics and injections);
- special diets, physical exercises that need to be taken to rehabilitate after an illness or operation;
- advice on diet and self-administering of injections of insulin for diabetic patients;
- explaining in advance details of an operation in order to reduce patient's anxiety;

- advice for persons diagnosed to be suffering from an illness, e.g. sickle cell anaemia, diabetes etc.;
- explaining to the parents of a dehydrated child how to prepare and give their child oral rehydration solution;
- advice on accompanying behaviour changes that are needed to control disease in the community, e.g. on use of condoms, safer sex, notification of partners when treating patients with sexually transmitted infections.

A well-organised patient education programme can speed up the recovery process, enable a hospital to discharge patients more quickly, release hospital beds and reduce complications and the need for follow-up.

There are many examples of health problems that could have been prevented with an effective patient education. One good example of the need for patient education is tuberculosis. A person must continue to take medicines for at least 6 months. Many stop taking medicines once they feel better and then the tuberculosis returns.

Another example of a patient education programme is a nutrition rehabilitation centre where, following diagnosis of malnutrition, the mother is allowed to stay with the child in the hospital. During the child's recovery she is given practical advice on nutrition and child feeding to prevent the child becoming malnourished again.

Growth monitoring is more than just the regular weighing of children and the detection of slowing of growth. The real importance of growth monitoring is, not the weighing itself, but the opportunity provided for education of parents about health, nutrition and child development.

Despite the importance of patient education it is often left out or not done very well. Health workers may not see the importance of it, they may feel that they have too many patients and do not have the time to give advice, they may think that they are already doing it but not realise that they are not being effective.

The standard patient education approach in many health settings – the 'health talk' – is often not done very well. It can suffer from many problems: noisy surroundings, too many people in the audience, not enough discussion, no visual aids and a general resentment by patients who may feel that they are being kept waiting when they want to see a health worker.

It is important to improve the quantity and quality of education provided during contact with patients. Pressure on doctors and nurses can be heavy and they may not have the time. Alternative approaches can include involving other support staff, e.g. pharmacists, dressers and volunteers, in patient education and holding special group teaching sessions, e.g. an oral rehydration corner, displays etc. For example the Baragwanath Hopital in Soweto, South Africa, developed a series of videos that could be shown while people were waiting. In the South Indian State of Tamil Nadu a project developed a series of audiocassettes with songs and drama on a range of health topics including nutrition and worms. Other ways for using waiting areas for patient education include: exhibitions, tables with leaflets on different topics and a library of books on self-care and health that can be borrowed by patients (see Figure 5.9).

The impact of patient education can be greatly increased through well-designed packaging in which the pills are set out in an easy to use way with clear instructions on their use. One of the best known examples of packaging is the 'blister' packaging of the oral contraceptive pill by which the daily dose is laid out in a way that it is easy to follow. This example has been followed by other medicines where the pills are set out on the pack according to dose. Clear instructions should be included using pictures on the packets or in accompanying leaflets. Pictures are especially useful for communities who cannot read but, as discussed in Chapter 3, it is very important to pre-test the words and pictures to make sure that they are understood.

In many communities people may go directly to shopkeepers and pharmacists for medicines. A valuable strategy used successfully for oral rehydration and malaria programmes has been to train pharmacists and shopkeepers so that they will be able to give proper advice on the use of medicines.

Packaging using childproof containers can also protect against the risk of accidental poison-

ing of children who may think medicines are sweets and eat them by mistake.

Solving these problems involves a planned approach to patient education. This involves carefully choosing the content to be relevant to the audience, providing support through training and supply of visual aids and appropriate packaging of medicines. Some of the steps in planning a patient education programme are listed on page 102.

Reorienting health services to promote health

In order to maximise the potential of health settings for the promotion of health you may need to improve the organisation and delivery of services. This may involve creating opportunities for education of patients, setting aside special areas for health education, providing a crèche where the children can be looked after for a short period while the mothers attend the patient-education session, improving provisions such as sanitation, water and meals.

According to WHO up to 75% of antibiotics are prescribed inappropriately resulting in ineffective treatment and growing antibiotic resistance. A response has been to seek to train health workers and pharmacists in improved prescribing practices.

The Health Promoting Hospital movement was launched by WHO in 1991 in Budapest in Hungary. While the initial focus was Europe, it is now spreading to other countries. In order to qualify for membership a hospital has to agree to implement a policy to promote the health and well-being of its patients and staff and to take a wider responsibility for the health of the surrounding community. Typical activities carried out by health promoting hospitals include patient education, training of staff in health education, providing healthy food in canteens, having a non-smoking policy, counselling and support services for staff and patients and setting up of outreach programmes in the community.

Another example of how services can be improved is the Baby Friendly Hospital Initiative to promote breastfeeding. Maternity hospitals

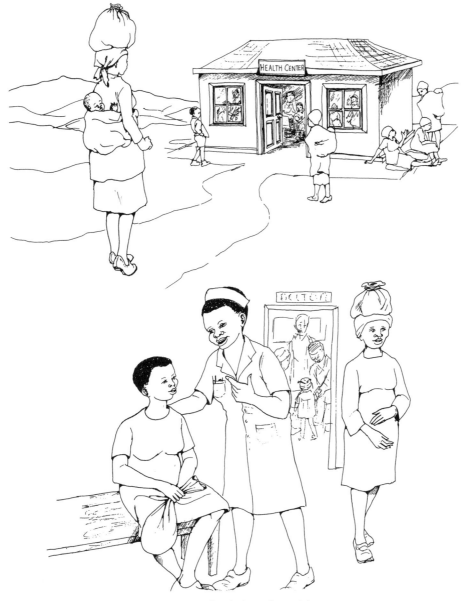

one-to-one
demonstrations
small-group sessions
self-help groups
lay health educators
drama and puppet shows
songs

wall-paintings (murals)
posters
real objects, e.g. foods, improved latrines
audiocassettes/videos in waiting areas
leaflets
lending libraries

**have all been used in health care settings
for patient-education**

Fig. 5.9   Patient education

Steps involved in planning a patient education programme

1. Find out what your intended audience thinks and feels about the health issue. You can apply the concepts introduced in Chapter 2 and identify: important beliefs and the role of culture; whether there are others in the family or community who should be involved in the patient education; and whether there are enabling factors such as resources or specific skills that have to be considered.
2. Identify and separate the different learning components of the patient education including: what facts need to be explained; the role of decision-making, psychomotor or communication skills; and whether there are any attitudes that should be encouraged, e.g. a positive attitude towards recovery and confidence in one's own ability to cope.
3. Apply the understandings gained in the two steps above and select the most appropriate advice to give (remember the characteristics of good advice given in Figure 3.6).
4. Decide *where* the patient education should take place: in the waiting area, during the consultation, after the consultation, in the hospital ward, or at the home of the patient?
5. Decide *who* should do the patient education – a doctor, nurse, lay counsellor or community health worker, pharmacist?
6. Decide what *method* to use – one-to-one, small group or large meeting; demonstrations, songs, puppet or theatre?
7. Decide what *learning aids* would be required to support the programme – real objects, models; wallcharts, flip chart, video; 'take home' reminders such as a leaflet or calendar?
8. Review the packaging of any drugs. If necessary change the packaging and instructions so that they are easier to follow and clear.
9. Decide how you will *evaluate* the outcome of the patient education in the short- and long-term.

Case studies of patient education programmes

A baby-friendly hospital programme in Bihar, North India. Doctors, nurses, and midwives at a district hospital were provided with a 10-day training course that explained the benefits and feasibility of early breastfeeding together with sessions on how to teach this information to mothers. Evaluation found that mothers who had received health education from the participating hospital were significantly more likely than mothers at a comparison hospital to breastfeed early. However, the evaluation pointed to the need for regular refresher training of staff to ensure that they continued to provide health education.

Programme to prevent the overuse of injections in a rural area near Yogyakarta, Indonesia. A single group discussion session with six patients and prescribers was held. The session lasted 90–120 minutes and was held in a relaxed informal setting of a restaurant with a free meal provided. The session included discussions of the prescribers' and patients' beliefs and motivations for injection use, the presentation of scientific materials and a conclusion. An evaluation found that, compared with patients at clinics not receiving the intervention, the programme had reduced use of injections from 70% to 42%. Injections of analgesics and vitamins almost halved. There was also a significant reduction in average number of drugs per prescription.

Two methods of advising mothers on infant feeding in Lima, Peru. The first intervention group of 70 received a recipe pamphlet and individual counselling on infant nutrition, especially the benefit of adding oil to weaning foods and of continued feeding of a baby with diarrhoea. The second intervention group of 70 received the same counselling and recipe book but also observed a cooking demonstration which lasted about 20 minutes. Both approaches improved the knowledge and practices of mothers to the same extent, showing that a simpler (and therefore cheaper!) method can sometimes be just as effective!

Patient education of surgery patients in a Nigerian hospital. Counselling was provided to patients before undergoing the following operations: laparotomy, colporrhaphy, herniorrhaphy and haemorrhoidectomy. Patients receiving counselling needed fewer painkillers and showed reduced anxiety levels when compared with patients who did not receive counselling.

Partner notification programme for sexually transmitted disease patients at an urban health centre in Lusaka, Zambia. One-to-one counselling lasting 10–20 minutes was provided for patients at a STD clinic. Female nurses talked with women patients and a male clinical officer talked to males. The counselling included information about STDs, the need to complete treatment, not having sex during treatment period and why and how they should inform their sexual partners. Patients received contact slips to give to all their sex partners. A follow-up study showed that more partners of the counselled patients were reached compared with a second group of patients who just received routine STD care.

A workplace based HIV/AIDS counselling among truck drivers in Kenya. Health workers and a health educator carried out informal group discussions, pre- and post-HIV test counselling and condom promotion at weekly clinics set up in depots of six of the largest trucking companies in Mombasa. Significant declines in self-reported high-risk sexual behaviour were found during a 1-year follow-up including reduction in extra-marital sex and use of sex workers. There was also a decrease in incidence of sexually transmitted infections.

Visual aids for patient education in rural Cameroon. Culturally-sensitive, visual aids were designed to convey instructions for use of prescription antibiotics (to illiterate women). The education involved use of visual aids and an 'advanced organiser'. The advanced organiser (introductory information used to explain why the drug is needed) used the example of farming to explain antibiotic use – a body as a crop field, disease as weeds, and antibiotics as a farmer. Pictures were based on photographs selected by the community as depicting local relevant scenes and were carefully pre-tested. An evaluation found that use of visual aids resulted in higher comprehension and adherence to the prescribed

antibiotics and that even more impact was achieved when using the advanced organiser.

Patient education of TB clinic in Cape Town, South Africa. Nurses were trained to counsel TB patients so that they would understand the treatment process and the importance of adhering to the full course of medicines. The patients were given a calendar on which they could mark their progress during treatment and gain a feeling of control over their own treatment. They were also given a picture storybook about a woman with TB who faced many obstacles to adherence, which included the shame and stigma of the disease, the depression she felt and the side effects of the medicines. She overcame those obstacles and was cured. The patients exposed to the educational input achieved a mean adherence rate to treatment of 95% with only one patient defaulting. A similar clinic that did not have the intervention had a lower mean adherence rate of 83% with 13 patients dropping out.

Patient education on diabetes in a hospital in Sri Lanka. The educational sessions consisted of talks by trained nurses, individual education, information leaflets and group discussions. This was reinforced at 2–3-month intervals by further education sessions by the nurses. The patients attending the diabetic clinic showed significant improvement in both knowledge and mean fasting blood glucose at 6 months compared with patients who did not receive the sessions.

wishing to join this movement agree to put into practice a programme of health education and reorientation of services. Further details of this are provided in Chapter 10.

Teaching and learning face-to-face communication skills

Most of the health education and health promotion programmes you undertake will involve some face-to-face communication activities. If you are involving field staff and volunteers you will probably need to include some training in face-to-face communication. Chapter 4 describes how you can prepare a job description followed up by a task analysis identifying the different kinds of learning involved including:

- any *facts* that should be learnt in order to give advice and make decisions;
- how to make any *decisions* required, e.g. planning the patient education or counselling programme, when to refer the client, e.g. for a HIV test, how to respond to difficult questions;
- face-to-face *communication skills* including listening skills, non-verbal communication, asking questions, obtaining feedback, showing empathy, using learning aids;
- *psychomotor skills* involved in the face-to-face encounter such as giving an injection, mixing a weaning food;
- *attitudes* especially respect, confidentiality, tolerance, patience.

One of the best ways of learning communication skills is through role-play where the participants act out the one-to-one or group situations and afterwards discuss and learn from their experiences. This can be followed up with practice in real situations in the community under supervision. The use of role-play methods is described in Chapter 4.

Summary

This chapter has looked at ways in which you can improve the effectiveness of your face-to-face communication skills.

1 Both verbal and non-verbal communication have an impact on the effectiveness of face-to-face encounters.
2 Listening is an active process involving asking questions and showing interest and responsiveness.
3 The effectiveness of face-to-face communication depends both on the choosing the right time and place for the encounter as well as

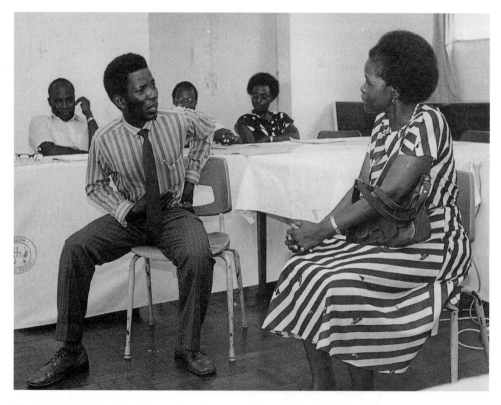

Fig. 5.10   Training health workers in counselling on AIDS in Uganda

good communication skills during the actual session.

4 Patient education should take into account principles of effective face-to-face communication, teaching and learning.

5 Patient education should be supported by improvements in health services including improvements in confidentiality, quality of case management, packaging of medicines, and creation of quiet areas.

6 Opportunities should be provided for field-workers to learn skills in face-to-face communication. The best way to acquire these skills is through role-play followed by practice under supervision in real-life situations.

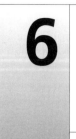

6 Working with communities

In earlier chapters you saw that many influences on people's behaviour are at the community level. Yet, in the past health educators have placed too much emphasis on health education with individuals in isolation from their family and community. Many difficulties people face in improving their health, such as poverty, lack of resources and exploitation by others, can only be overcome if people work together for their common good.

The introductory chapter of this book described different approaches to health education. The persuasion approach was contrasted with a health empowerment approach emphasising community participation and empowerment. When the idea of primary health care was launched, community participation was one of the most important components. Community participation was also part of the more recent idea of health promotion. But community participation is a term that is not understood very well. Although everyone talks about it, community participation is often not put into practice. This chapter will explore different ways of working at the community level for the promotion of health. In particular it will:

1 Explain the concept of community participation, its difference from the conventional 'top down' planning approaches and the advantages that can come from involving communities in participating in health education programmes.

2 Explore the difficulties encountered in community participation programmes and how these problems can be resolved by careful planning.
3 Examine the role of communication and participatory learning methods in working for change at the community level.

Concept of community participation

The first question that we need to consider is, what does community participation really mean? What do we mean by the community becoming involved and participating in improvement of health?

The word community is used in many different ways. It can be used to describe: a *place* or small geographical area; a *group* of people sharing some interest; or a *social network* of relationships at a local level. So 'community' means more than just people who live close together, it implies sharing and working together in some way. As you will see in a later section, people can live in the same village, but be divided in interests and share little in common.

The term community can also be applied to people who do not live in the same neighbourhood but share characteristics, e.g. youths, sex workers, an ethnic minority, drug addicts, people with disabilities. An *outreach approach* is the name that is sometimes used for educational programmes directed at a special group that do not necessarily live in the same neighbourhood.

'Top-down' and 'bottom-up' approaches

One way of defining community participation is to compare it with other approaches that do not involve participation. The traditional approach in health care planning is for the decisions to be made by senior persons in health services – the so-called 'experts'. This approach is sometimes called the 'top-down' approach and contrasted with the 'bottom-up' approach where members of the community make the decisions.

This approach of leaving decisions to professional persons is also used by many health educators. Research may be carried out through surveys to find out what the community thinks and believes to be the problems. But in the end it is usually the health educator who makes the decisions on what goes into the programmes based on medically-defined needs.

Traditional education is often *indoctrination*. Indoctrination is the process of telling people what to do. We make the decisions and expect them to follow. Many people assume that just

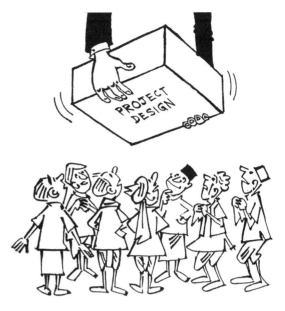

Fig. 6.1   A top-down approach to planning

because they have invited members of the community to a meeting, community participation is taking place. This is not always the case and you will need to look carefully to find out what is really going on. Are the planners using it just to

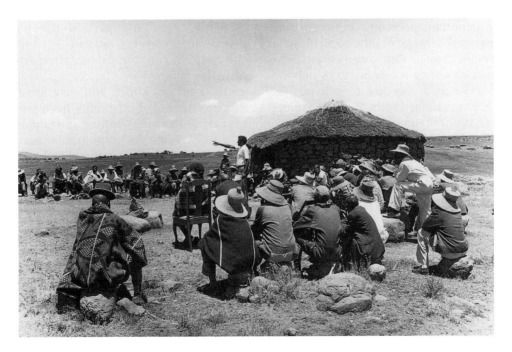

Fig. 6.2   Just because there is a meeting does not mean there is community participation

tell the villagers what to do? Or have they come to consult the people and give them a say in their own future?

The term community participation is often applied to programmes where self-help labour is used. The community may contribute their labour to dig a latrine for the school in their village. However, is this genuine participation? Are they doing it because they have been told to do it? Or did they decide themselves to do it?

Spectrum of participation

When we carefully examine different interpretations of the phrase 'community participation' we find that it is used to cover a whole range of very different actions. The American planner Sherry Arnstein suggested that there is a continuum of participation (Figure 6.3). At one extreme there are actions that are really forms of manipulation. Manipulation means controlling people like puppets even though we pretend to let them make decisions.

At the opposite extreme there is total participation or complete control of their affairs by the community. For example we may give the local community control over the health budget for a locality. They may run the health clinic and make the important decisions. Between these two extremes are a range of other activities that can sometimes happen. One common activity is consultation or asking a community's opinion. However, holding a meeting to ask people's opinions is a very limited form of participation if the final decisions are made by outsiders.

An outreach programme usually involves sending fieldworkers into communities to work with people who have particular needs – such as young people or drug addicts, etc. The fieldworkers can be health workers or recruited from the target communities themselves. An outreach approach can be top-down when all the decision-making and priorities are set by the external agency. However it is also possible to use a community participation approach if the target communities and locally recruited field workers are allowed to participate in decision-making.

Projects may say that they are using community participation or involvement and it is important to find out whether this is actually true. David Werner sees community participation as one of the key features that distinguish what he calls 'community supportive' from 'community oppressive' programmes. The list below draws on the work of David Werner, Susan Rifkin and Patricia Martin and presents a checklist of questions you can apply to find out how much participation is really taking place.

What benefits come from community participation?

Many people find it unnecessary to justify community participation. They see it as a fundamental right and part of the process of democracy. However, as you will see later in the chapter, genuine community participation must be planned in advance and will require extra time and effort. You may need to convince others of the benefits from community participation to get funding and support.

Justifications for community participation come from a variety of sources including lessons learned from the failures of conventional 'top-down' educational programmes as well as the achievements of community-based programmes.

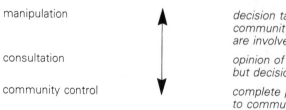

Fig. 6.3   Simplified version of Arnstein's ladder of participation

A checklist of questions for finding the degree of participation in a programme
• Is the community involved in planning, management and control of the health programme at the community level?
• Were the felt needs of the community found out at the outset of the programme and was notice taken of them in planning the programme objectives?
• What forms of social organisation exist in the community and to what extent have they been involved in the decision-making process such as farmers' cooperatives, clubs, churches, political organisations and trade unions?
• Is there a mechanism for dialogue between health system personnel and community leadership?
• Is there a mechanism for community representatives to be involved in decision-making at higher levels and is this effective?
• Is there any evidence of the external agents changing their plans as a result of criticism from the community?
• Are deprived groups such as the poor, landless, unemployed and women adequately represented in the decision-making process?
• Are local resources used, e.g. labour, buildings money?
• Was the community involved in evaluating the project and in drafting of the final report?

Types of community groups	
Self-help groups	Run by people for their own benefit such as cooperatives and stop smoking groups (see discussion of self-help groups in previous chapter).
Representative groups	Elected and answerable to the community – e.g. community associations.
Pressure groups	A group of self-appointed citizens taking action on what they see to be the interests of the whole community – such as putting pressure to improve the school, get garbage collected, do something about a dangerous road.
Traditional organisations	Well-established groups usually meeting the needs of a particular section of the community such as: Rotary Club, mothers' union, parent–teacher association, church group.
Social groups	Exist mainly to put on social events, e.g. sports clubs, music groups, carnival group.
Welfare groups	Exist to improve welfare for others, e.g. run feeding programmes.

The need for a community approach

An important justification for community participation is the need to shift the emphasis from the individual to the community. In earlier chapters you will have seen that many influences on a behaviour are at the community level and not under the control of individuals. These include social pressure from other people through norms, shared culture and the local socio-economic situation. Even when the influences are at the national level, it is often through pressure from communities that governments will make changes.

The list below describes some of the different kinds of groups that you might already find in the community or may start up yourself as a result of your community participation programme.

Drawing on local knowledge

Communities often have detailed knowledge about their surroundings. This 'community environmental knowledge' includes the plants, animals, water sources, building materials, and treatment and prevention of disease. It makes sense to involve communities in making plans because they know local conditions and the possibilities for change.

Making programmes locally relevant and acceptable

A major problem in the development of health services is the gap between the decision-makers and the community. A common complaint is that their projects are not supported and maintained by the community. However, usually the community was never consulted. If the community is involved in choosing priorities and deciding on plans, people are much more likely to become involved in the programme and take up the services because they see the programme to be meeting their needs. The timings and location will be more appropriate to the community who will then be more likely to use them.

A good example of the importance of community participation comes from the experiences of water-supply programmes where the community can participate in: choosing the best location of water taps; providing labour in the initial construction; ensuring that the water systems are used properly; and in setting up a community organisation for reporting breakdowns and carrying out simple maintenance. The cartoons in this chapter are all taken from The World Health Organization's excellent manual *Achieving Success in Water and Sanitation*.

Developing self-reliance, self-confidence, empowerment and problem-solving skills

The enthusiasm that comes from community participation can lead to a greater sense of

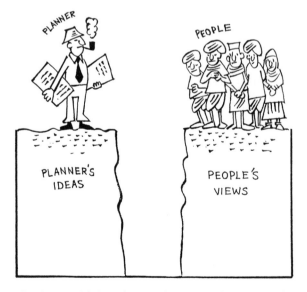

Fig. 6.4   Bridging the gap between planners and the community

self-reliance for the future. For example – communities are usually willing to participate in water programmes because they see that benefits will come. The feeling of community solidarity and self-reliance from participating in decisions over their own future through a water project can lead to further activities.

Better relationship between health worker and community

Community participation leads to a better relationship between the community and health workers. Instead of a servant–master relationship, there is trust and partnership.

Primary health care

The Alma Ata Declaration on Primary Health Care in 1978 extended the notion of appropriate health care beyond that of simply providing decentralised services. It also considered the need to tackle economic and social causes of ill health. Health education and community participation are essential (and often missing!) ingredients of primary health care.

The beneficial effects of social networks and social capital

In Chapter 2 the concept of social networks was introduced to describe the relationship of people with each other in communities. You saw how the influence of other people can lead a person to act in a specific way. Social networks were also discussed in Chapter 3 as channels through which people receive information and new ideas about the world around them – the internal communication system. Alongside social pressure and information sources, social networks have a third important function – the provision of care and support. The family and community play an important role in care and support in bringing up families, and in times of crisis such as sickness, bereavement, unemployment, disasters. The nature and extent of social networks can change from society to society and extend from the couple, parents and children, grandparents, other relatives and involve the whole community.

The importance of economic capital – income and wealth – in tackling poverty and inequalities in health has long been recognised. However, in recent years a greater awareness of the beneficial role of social networks has led to the introduction of the concept of 'social capital' by agencies such as the World Bank, who define it as 'the institutions, relationships, and norms that shape the quality and quantity of a society's social interactions…social capital is not just the sum of the institutions which underpin a society – it is the glue that holds them together.' Indicators that have been used to measure social capital have included measures such as the amount of volunteering that takes place, community support structures, community trust in civil organisations, absence of violence and crime. While the concept of social capital is widely accepted, there is less agreement on the specifics, which will vary from culture to culture.

Anything that affects the functioning of communities can affect social networks and social capital. Poverty, war, cultural invasion of foreign practices, growth of cities and diseases such as AIDS are among the many factors that cause fragmentation of communities through death of family members, forced migration to cities in search of work and displacement to refugee camps. Where strong social networks already exist, community participation programmes need to build upon those existing structures. Where networks are weak and fragmented, community participation programmes should create social capital by working to build up trust, cooperation, community organisation and joint action.

Benefits of community participation

Emphasises community rather than individuals.
Makes programmes relevant to local situation.
Ensures community motivation and support.
Improves take-up of services.
Promotes self-help and self-reliance.
Improves communication between health workers and community.
Enables the development of primary health care.
Strengthens social networks and social capital.

Case studies of community-based health promotion activities

Community-based distribution of malaria prophylaxis in Central Java. Ten persons from each of three villages were trained to distribute chloroquine to prevent malaria. Each person visited 20 households per week to detect fever, take blood and give health education. After the intervention the spleen rates, parasite rates and fever cases dropped to nearly zero.

Using mobile units to promote uptake of screening for cervical cancer in a rural district in Thailand. Mobile units visited health centres and village primary schools to take cervical smears free of charge. Health information about cervical cancer and the importance of the screening was disseminated to the villages through radio, village loudspeakers and leaflets. A few days before the mobile unit was due to arrive an evening group lecture and discussion was given to the village health communicators and adult women in each village. The village health communicators were asked to give health education to any woman in their community who might not have received the health information and to invite them personally to the screening programme. Surveys of the target community found that the knowledge of the importance of cervical cancer increased and that the proportion of women who had been screened rose from 20% to almost 60%.

AIDS education in cattle markets and festivals in North East Thailand. At weekly cattle markets cattle market managers and the owners of the food shops were involved. A wide range of educational media were developed including: messages on condom boxes, T-shirts for food vendors, posters and hanging mobiles for shops, stickers for trucks and motorcycles and key chains with pull-out drawers for condoms. Condoms were provided free. At the festivals, which took place at special occasions such as the Thai New Year, village health workers were involved. Competitions were held for songs and the winning songs distributed on cassettes for broadcasts on village loudspeakers. A 2-month follow-up found that many people had been exposed to the educational messages, there was a greater willingness of clients to use condoms with sex workers and increased sales of condoms from shops.

Outreach home-visiting programme to support breastfeeding in Mexico City. Persons aged 25–30 years were trained to give home-based counselling through a combination of classes, demonstration and observation/work experience at lactation clinics and mother-to-mother support groups. A follow-up study of mothers 3 months after delivery found that exclusive breastfeeding was practised by 67% of mothers who had been visited six times by the outreach workers and by 50% of the mothers who were visited three times. Of a group of mothers who were not visited by outreach workers, only 12% practised exclusive breastfeeding.

Involving shopkeepers in Kenya in malaria control. A total of 43 shopkeepers were trained in a series of three 3-day workshops to use two types of materials to give correct information to purchasers on the use of chloroquine and aspirin/paracetamol-based drugs. Two visual aids were developed: a chart to help the shopkeeper determine correct dosage and a set of rubber stamps to print out information for the purchaser showing the correct way of using chloroquine for children. An evaluation found that the percentage of childhood fevers where an adequate dose of chloroquine was given to the child rose from only 4% before the training to 65% after training.

Promoting birth spacing among the Maya-Quiché of Guatemala. The 3-year campaign consisted of health education supported by: (1) improvements in quality of services through training, supervisory visits and continuous supply of contraceptives and recruitment of volunteer promoters; and (2) inter-sectoral collaboration with other development agencies. The health education consisted of a national television messages directed at the whole population and media specifically designed for this illiterate Mayan community – including two radio spots, a vehicle-mounted loudspeaker for the market place and other community settings, and a video produced in the local language for showing at meetings and for

triggering discussions. An evaluation found that contraceptive use rose from 5% to 18% over the 3-year period.

A village-based intervention to prevent HIV/AIDS in Thailand. The intervention consisted of three parts: (1) a meeting with village leaders followed by selection and training of volunteer leaders from the village to act as facilitators; (2) broadcasts from village loudspeakers over 5 days of an audio-drama and display of 10 posters depicting each day's major issues – the plot of the drama revolved around married men engaging commercial sex workers, risk reduction strategies, and dialogues between women, between spouses and between men; (3) a village meeting to discuss the drama and plan further. The evaluation found that village meetings were widely attended, both men and women responded positively to the audio-drama, perceptions about HIV/AIDS changed and that women were more likely to recognise that they were personally at risk as a result of their husband going with sex workers.

Concept of needs

Before proceeding further, we need to examine critically the concept of needs and the implications this has for the process of community participation. Basing a health programme on a community's felt needs is often criticised by planners and health workers. They often object and claim that the members of the community are not really able to define their own needs. However this raises fundamental questions. What do we mean by needs? In reality, there is no such thing as the 'real need' for a particular community but a range of perspectives.

- ***Felt needs*** are what people 'feel' or their 'wants'. They may only be the feelings of individual people or a collective feeling shared by the whole group.
- ***Expressed needs*** have not only been felt but have been brought to the attention of the authorities – i.e. 'expressed' – by requests, petitions or complaints.
- ***Agency-determined needs*** are what external services such as health workers and planners

have decided that the community need. They do not necessarily correspond to felt needs.

Many 'community participation' programmes are really 'top-down' and based on agency-determined needs. However, imposing our views on communities is dangerous because we do not always understand the whole situation. It also represents a rejection of the community's right to determine their own needs. Also, if the community has strongly held felt needs, it is unlikely to take action on the agency-determined needs.

Felt needs are based on people's judgements of their present situation and possibilities for change. These judgements may depend on beliefs about the extent and nature of health problems, their causes and possibilities for prevention and cure. These beliefs are influenced by their previous experience, education, understanding of biology and causes of disease. So felt needs may be based on a realistic assessment of their situation by the community. But they can also be based on misunderstandings and incomplete knowledge.

For example, many communities think of health as a product of doctors and medicines. They are more likely to define their felt needs in terms of wanting health facilities and curative services rather than preventive measures.

- *Felt needs* include a person's or community's assessment of the present situation and potential for change;
- *which may depend on beliefs* about the extent and nature of health problems, their causes and possibilities for prevention and cure; and
- *are influenced by previous experience*, culture, education understanding of epidemiology and biology.

Another problem in community participation comes with the concept of community itself. We often assume that everyone in a village or community agrees with each other and shares the same felt needs. This is not always the case. Societies may be divided according to inequalities in wealth, power and employment. This is called 'social stratification' (literally the 'layering' of the community). Other forms of divisions can exist according to religion, language, tribe or race.

People may disagree with each other. It can be very difficult to get everyone to agree at public meetings over what they want. Frequently the needs that emerge from meetings

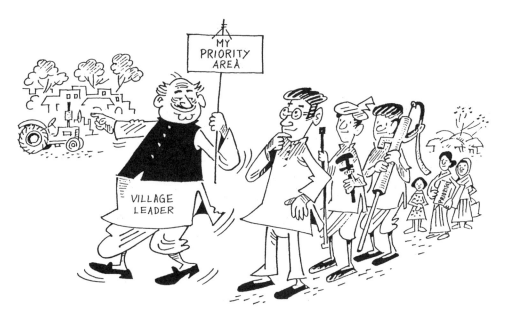

Fig. 6.5   You can easily be misled if you do not understand the divisions in a community

are those of the dominant powerful groups. The needs of disadvantaged sections of the community, such the poor or women, may be ignored. For example, a recent review of community participation in family planning projects in Asia describes how the various local committees consisted mainly of male elders. A criticism of the nationwide community development programme set up in India in the 1950s is that village 'panchayat' committees were dominated by high-caste, landowning, and better-off men.

So community participation is not simply a passive process of responding to needs of the community but an *active process* of working with groups to define needs. This should be based on dialogue, sharing of understandings and ensuring that the needs that are acted upon are based on informed decision-making and represent the interests of all sections of the community. This process of dialogue is shown in Figure 6.6, which is loosely based on the work of Batten.

Community participation as a process

Community participation cannot be achieved through occasional visits and holding meetings. You should allow a realistic timescale for your programme. It should be seen as a *process* over time that can go through a series of overlapping stages such as those shown in Figure 6.7.

Entry: getting to know the community

The starting point for any community-based activity is to get to know the community. You will need to identify and have informal discussion with opinion leaders, community groups, fieldworkers from government and non-governmental organisations. It is helpful to make a *profile* of the community in order to identify any special features that will affect the success of community participation programmes. It is important to know of any previous health programmes that may have taken place in that area – and whether they were successes or failures.

You should try to discover the felt needs of the community. It may have already brought some of them to the attention of heath and other services through complaints and letters. If not, you will have to meet individuals and groups to find out their felt needs. It is important to know whether the whole community agrees on the needs or if there are differences. Are there minorities with different needs? Are there conflicting interests?

Listed here is a range of different types of information that you might find useful in planning your programme. The data required will

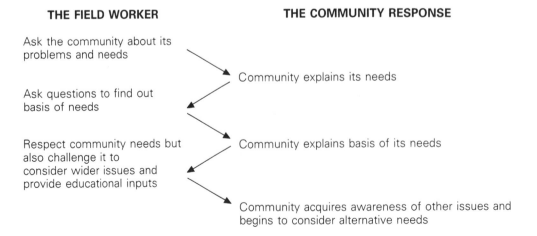

Fig. 6.6   The process of dialogue in community participation

Entry: getting to know the community

↓

Initial actions

↓

Further activities and
organisation-building

↓

Evaluation and reflection

*Learning about the community, its
structure and pattern; initial contacts
with families, leaders and community
groups; discussions on concerns and felt
needs.*

*Action on achievable, short-term aims
based on felt needs which bring the
community together and build
confidence.*

*Strengthening of community
organisation; formation of committees;
educational inputs; selection of
community members for training as lay
workers; decision-making on priorities;
further actions.*

*Reflection on achievements; decisions
about future activities; reduction in
dependence on external project and
greater community involvement in future
activities.*

Fig. 6.7   Stages in community participation programmes

depend on the health issues you are interested in, and the special features of the locality. You should also consult with the community themselves over the type of information to collect.

In any community there will always be individuals with special influence. These opinion leaders may be chiefs, religious leaders, teachers or older persons. It is important to find out who are the opinion leaders and what *they* think are the needs of the community. They can help you in many ways – but beware of being misled (see Figure 6.5)!

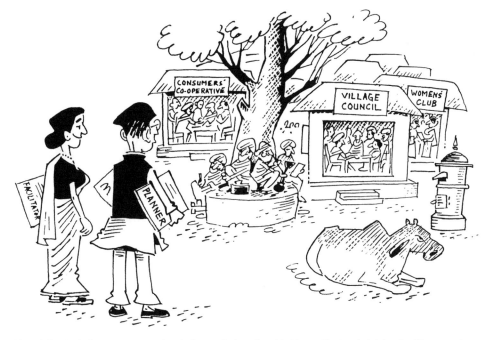

Fig. 6.8   It is important to look for existing institutions that might be built upon in community participation programmes

Information required for making the community profile

Environment: geography, urban/rural, transport, land use, recreational facilities, housing.

History: history of area, activities of local groups, issues that the community have expressed concern about in the past; previous government and NGO activities on health; previous history of community action.

General data: total population, age distribution, children under 14 years, population 65 years, under-fives, turnover of population, birth rate, family sizes, vulnerable groups such as single-parent families, people with disabilities, ethnic groups, religion, social class, employment.

Health and other services: utilisation of hospitals/clinics/private doctors, traditional healers; social services, agriculture, community development, adult education, schools; other government services; relationships with community and other agencies; degree of conflict and cooperation between agencies.

Perceptions of area: residents' perceptions of problems of area; attitudes towards other residents, agencies, officials, local politicians, attitudes and beliefs concerning health and felt needs for health education and health care services.

Community structure, norms and traditions: networks of information, influence and care; family structure; opinion leaders, divisions and conflicts; power structure; norms that determine people's attitudes to taking action to achieve some change; norms that govern the role of women; norms that govern health and illness behaviour.

Organisations: religious organisations; women's groups, youth groups, non-governmental organisations.

Communications: local newspapers, newsletter, notice boards, radio, television.

Power and leadership: existing community organisations, committees etc., businesses; trade unions; elected politicians; political parties; local political forums such as ward councils; officials in health services, housing and education.

The contribution of local leaders to community health education

1. Bring people to meetings.
2. Arrange for and find meeting places.
3. Help reach more people by telling others.
4. Help people in the community know you and gain confidence in you.
5. Give general information about the programme and help interpret it to the people.
6. Help identify problems and resources in the community.
7. Help plan and organise programmes and community activities.
8. Help plan and organise any services that might be provided.
9. Give simple demonstrations.
10. Conduct meetings.
11. Lead youth groups and various individual projects.
12. Interest others in becoming leaders.
13. Help neighbours learn skills.
14. Share information with neighbours.
15. Serve as an officer in an organisation or chairperson of a committee.

(Adapted from Peace Corps (1978). *Community Health Education in Developing Countries – Getting Started*)

Initial actions

Building up community participation may involve meeting individuals to find out about the problems of the area. It also involves working with large groups. It is usual to have community meetings early in the programme. These provide an opportunity for everybody to participate in the discussion. But you should carefully prepare yourself to deal with questions and problems that might arise. Find out if people are going to bring up an issue, such as roads or the state of the local school, that is outside your own control. You can then invite persons from those departments to join in the discussion.

How you proceed will depend a great deal on the power structure of the community and the presence of divisions and opposing interests. Some of the ways communities can be split into factions are shown in Figure 6.9. How do you think your approach might differ with each of the community structures?

With only one faction in the community as in (1) you will need to work with that single group and its leader. With situations (2) and (3) where there are two or more factions it is more difficult and you will have to balance the needs of different groups and avoid appearing to favour one group over another. You will have to find areas of common interest on which the groups can agree.

Most rural communities will have well-developed social structures. However the situation in urban areas can be quite different and resemble (4). If there are no distinct groups, such as in a newly-created housing settlement your priority should be to encourage some kind of community structure to be developed. You can do this by finding an issue that everyone is concerned about enough to attend meetings and take action.

These early decisions on issues and actions will have an important influence on future developments. A successful outcome will build up confidence. You should encourage the community to select short-term achievable objectives that will unite different factions in common action.

Further activities and organisation building

The success of this initial action should result in the community seeing the benefits of working together, gaining more confidence and attracting more people to join in activities. The need for some structure will become apparent. Out of the large meeting, a small group is often formed, such as a village water committee. You can work closely with these small groups and advise them on the best way to organise themselves and help to resolve any internal tensions and conflicts.

As the community begins to develop trust and confidence in you, they will be prepared to listen to your suggestions for further actions. Individuals in the community will begin to acquire new skills as a result of their involvement and will identify needs for further education. You should continue your dialogue and provide educational inputs in response to their interests. As their perspectives broaden, they will be prepared to tackle wider issues. You should take a less active role and encourage the community to take more responsibility for maintaining the project.

	Community structure	Your response
(1)	One main group with single leader	Work with the single organisation and leader
(2)	Two groups (in this case one larger than the other)	Find point of agreement between the two groups
(3)	Community divided into more than two factions	Find point of agreement between the groups
(4)	No distinct structures or divisions (e.g. newly-occupied area which has not yet developed a social structure)	Identify issues that will encourage people to come together and encourage formation of community structures and emergence of leadership

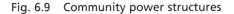

Fig. 6.9   Community power structures

Evaluation and reflection

As activities progress, you should be keeping a record of achievements so you can evaluate the programme. The local community can share in the evaluation of the programme through collecting data and providing support for survey teams. Results of any evaluation can be discussed with the community, who should be given an opportunity to reflect on their achievements and share in the making of longer-term plans for their area.

The big test for any community participation programme is whether activities continue once external support is reduced. Activities will continue or collapse depending on the strength of the community structures created during the early activities.

These stages, described above, should not be applied in a rigid way. They should be seen as overlapping components of a process of working with communities. Whether or not you have to go through them depends on the situation in the community and what has already happened. In some situations there will already be a range of community-based activities that you can build upon. In other communities there be few activities and divisions or conflicts and you need to start by building up community organisation.

Participatory learning and education for critical awareness

It is important to build learning experiences into community participation programmes. In this way, the community will be able to understand more about the different factors that influence their health and how these factors can be changed. But the approach to teaching should be quite different from traditional health education where the teacher is the 'expert' and the community is expected to accept what it is told and often made to feel inferior. It is important to use methods that develop a critical awareness of the situation and *empower* the community to work together for change.

The Brazilian adult educator/priest Paulo Freire has been an influential critic of traditional formal educational approaches. He was deeply critical of traditional approaches to education, which he compared with depositing facts in people's heads, rather like money in a bank. Instead, he calls for a problem-posing approach involving dialogue on an equal basis between the community and the educator.

> In problem-posing education people develop their power to perceive critically the way they exist in the world with which and in which they find themselves; they come to see the world not as a static reality but as a reality in process, in transformation.
>
> Paulo Freire

The special name he uses for this approach to education is '*conscientisation*' or consciousness-raising. In this approach, the community is encouraged to *reflect* critically on their situation and how they might transform it through action. The process of learning from action he called 'praxis'.

Participatory learning methods have already been discussed in Chapter 4 and characteristics of educational methods for promoting empowerment are shown here, adapted from the work of Susan Kindervatter.

Paulo Freire's method was to prepare pictures of every-day situations and difficulties. These were shown to the community who were then asked to discuss and critically reflect on

---

Characteristics of learning methods for empowerment

- Opportunities are built in for discussion, feedback and participation.
- Methods used usually involve simulations, role-plays and problem-solving exercises: learning aids such as flannelgraphs and pictures are used that can promote discussion.
- Less emphasis is put on acquisition of specific knowledge and more on development of problem-solving skills, critical thinking, reflection and analysis.
- Small groups (fewer than 20) are used.
- Learning is open-ended with objectives determined by the whole group.
- Trainer acts as facilitator to process rather than teacher and 'expert'.

them. Others, such as the Laedza Batanani Theatre Group in Botswana, have followed his approach using drama instead of pictures. In their programme, a theatre group visited communities and developed the drama from local issues. Following presentation of the drama, the community was involved in discussion of the issues and suggesting solutions. It was possible to stop the drama at different stages and ask for comments, suggestions or for the community to take part. Another approach is to use the community themselves as actors and let them base the content of the drama on their experiences. Chapter 7 will give more examples of theatre for community participation.

Many people are only used to traditional formal one-way teaching. They can find it threatening to have discussion and criticism in the session. So it is important to provide support through training in participatory learning methods to fieldworkers in community-based projects. *Training for Transformation* is a particularly useful set of manuals on participatory methods. Lyra Srinivasan of the non-governmental organisation World Education pioneered a set of participatory learning methods that were later adapted for use in nutrition education by Save the Children Fund and by the United Nations Development Programme PROWESS programme for use in water and sanitation and by Sue Laver and AIDS Action for use in education on AIDS. Some of the methods they introduce are described on the right.

Participatory rural appraisal

Understanding the community is vitally important for effective community participation. One of the most interesting developments in recent years has been the use of participatory rural appraisal method (PRA) – also called participatory learning and action (PLA). PRA is a tool for entering a community, involving people in examining their community and making decisions on action. The approach builds upon the ideas introduced by Paulo Freire who emphasised the importance of encouraging a community to reflect upon its situation and

---

Examples of participatory learning exercises

Discussion posters (also called picture codes). Pictures are used to trigger a discussion. The picture is shown to a group and the facilitator encourages discussion by asking questions: What do you see in this picture? What is the problem shown? How do you think it can be solved?

Activity exercises. A picture of a child is put on a wall and the community are asked to mark on the picture the signs they know of dehydration.

3-pile sorting cards. A set of pictures is produced showing practices that affect a particular health issue. The cards are given to the community who are asked to put them into three piles: those they consider to be good for health, those that are bad for health, and ones that they are not certain about. For example 3-pile sorting cards for education on HIV/AIDS might have pictures of condoms, people hugging, eating, about to have sex, sharing razors, shaking hands, caring for a person with HIV/AIDS. They are encouraged to discuss the reasons for their decisions.

Unserialised posters. The group is given a set of pictures and asked to put them into any order they like and to tell a story with them. Sequences of pictures that might be used could include a community with onchocerciasis, going for treatment, receiving treatment; or a person with a sexually transmitted disease, going to the clinic, breaking the news to a partner, returning with partner for treatment, taking the medicines and using condoms.

Story with a gap. The group is given two pictures – one showing a scene with actions that are harmful for heath and the other a scene when they have taken action to deal with the problem. The group is asked to make up a story about how the community moved from the health problem, e.g. problems of malaria breeding sites, poor water or rubbish, and took action to deal with it. In the discussion the group is asked to consider if similar actions could be taken to improve their community.

---

take action. PRA is a process of working with a community over a few days. During this period the community is encouraged to undertake a set of activities which includes those listed below. In carrying out these activities, communities embark on a process of describing their community, reflecting on their present status and considering priorities for change.

Some methods used in PRA

Transect walk. The facilitators and community walk through the village observing local practices and engaging the community in conversation about local conditions, needs and priorities.

Mapping. The community are encouraged to draw maps on the ground or large sheet of paper. The maps show the location of houses, features such as water sources, social relationships between community members etc.

Venn or chapatti diagrams or institutional maps. The community draw diagrams in which different groups and organisations in the community are represented by circles and their relationships and importance in decision-making are shown by the size of the circles and the extent to which they overlap.

Seasonal calendars. These are drawn on the ground with stones and other objects used to show facts such as rainfall, workload, busy times in the field, times when diseases are more common, times of food scarcity or when money is scarce. The calendar is useful for identifying times when the community is vulnerable or when opportunities present themselves for action.

Daily activity charts. The community show how they spend their day. This is useful for getting an idea of daily activities and divisions that exist in workload and risk by age, gender and other characteristics.

Problem ranking. One approach is to ask participants to list six main problems either in general or related to a specific area, e.g. health, and then to ask them to rank them in order of importance. Another way of doing this is through *pair-wise ranking* in which the facilitator prepares a card for each problem identified. The facilitator then shows the communities pairs of cards and asks 'which is the bigger problem?'. The final result is obtained by counting the number of times that each problem won over the others and arranging them in order of importance. Problem ranking is useful for bringing out felt needs of communities and different priorities between different sections of the community, e.g. young, elders, men and women.

Wealth ranking. Communities are involved in identifying and analysing different wealth groups in a community. This could be through asking a group to list the different families in their community and put them in order of wealth. This can also be done with names on cards or by representing different households by stones or other objects and placing them on different piles according to their wealth. Wealth ranking is useful for gaining an understanding of how the community look at wealth and divide up their community. Wealth is a very sensitive issue and wealth ranking may be difficult to carry out.

PRA has been widely used by programmes working in the field of environmental education, gender education, nutrition and health. The UK-based NGO – the International Institute for Environment and Development – has taken a lead role in the promotion of PRA as a tool for development.

PRA can provide many rich insights into a community. It is not only a research tool but a way of entering a community, engaging in dialogue and involving a larger and more representative group of the community through activities that are entertaining, fun but at the same time challenging. PRA bridges the gap between understanding the community and action. However, set against its many advantages there are some important considerations to take into account. You have to allow sufficient time for the process. You should not do PRA unless you are prepared to follow it up and work with communities to implement the actions they identify as important. At the same time you have to be careful not to raise expectations that you are unable to fulfil. The field staff who carry out the PRA should have the training and experience to negotiate the activities in the community and deal with any problems that may arise. In communities that are divided and in a state of conflict, some of the PRA activities will be very difficult – especially in such controversial areas such as problem ranking and wealth ranking.

Using lay workers and volunteers

Any information about health that you give the community will get passed on to others through informal contacts. We can deliberately encourage this process by selecting members of the community and giving them training as health educators. An approach that is now used in many primary health programmes is to encourage communities to select one of themselves to receive simple training as village health workers or community health workers. They can become highly effective communicators because they share the same background characteristics as their fellow villagers. The term *peer education* is used when the same approach is used for reaching sections of the community, such as sex workers, truck drivers, prisoners, out-of-school youths, or street children, who may be difficult to reach through other channels.

Two approaches have been used for selection of lay persons for training. In 'outreach' projects, the health education agency appoints the lay persons. They may have been selected as a result of having been identified as 'opinion leaders' or through a process such as advertising and recruiting from a public meeting. However, in programmes that emphasise community participation, it is best to ask the community to select one or more of their members for training as a lay health educator. With the expansion in interest in Primary Health Care there have been many experiments using community health workers and evaluations have suggested the guidelines shown here.

Planning for community participation

You have seen that community participation can bring considerable benefits to health programmes. However, overcoming the problems described above and achieving community participation requires careful planning.

Involvement of other sectors

The community may bring up needs that cannot be met by the health services. For example

---

Guidelines for using lay workers in community health programmes

- The persons selected should match the project's needs. If you are trying to reach youths, then train young people as 'peer educators'. If you are working with women, use women of a similar age to the target groups.
- Select people who are already respected in the community. They may be people who are leading figures in the community programmes, traditional birth attendants, traditional healers or other respected persons.
- Involve the community in the selection of the volunteers. Brief them on the kinds of personal qualities that are needed of trustworthiness, acceptability, skill as a communicator and educational background.
- Provide a training that is practical and includes participatory learning methods.
- Provide regular support and follow-up to encourage the volunteers in their work. Give them opportunities to share their problems with you and the other volunteers.

Tumwine described how he and his colleagues recognised a high incidence of schistosomiasis in a rural Zimbabwe village and were planning to motivate the community to build and use improved latrines. He asked the people what their main problems were. He expected the response 'schistosomiasis', but to his surprise, they answered 'food' and a disease whose description fitted pellagra. The team ended up discussing drought, relief food and food production.

If your own programme is not very flexible and cannot follow this example, it would be important to involve persons from other departments such as agriculture, rural development and adult literacy. If they are involved, they can act on social and economic needs and you can concentrate on meeting the felt needs that are specific to health. But health, social and economic needs all are interrelated so it is important that you work as a team.

If your activities only involve a single health topic such as AIDS, water, nutrition, sanitation

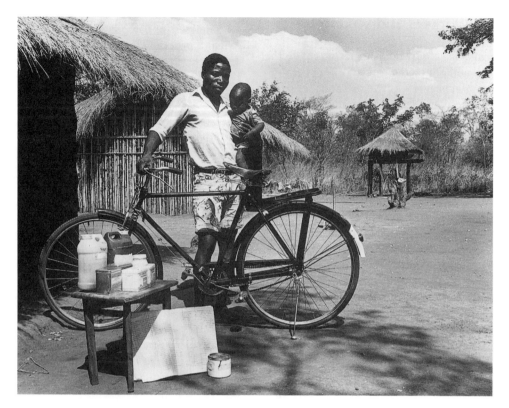

Fig. 6.10 Village health worker

Case studies of the use of lay workers and peer educators in health promotion

Involving partners of volunteers in Guatemala. A family planning experiment in Guatemala used community volunteers (called 'distributors'). Spouses of volunteers were provided with a 3-day training course on family planning and contraceptives. Volunteers whose spouses were involved were more effective at promoting contraception than those whose spouses were not involved.

Community-based distribution of malaria prophylaxis in Central Java, Indonesia. Ten people from each village were trained to distribute chloroquine as prophylaxis – each person visited 20 households per week to detect fever, take blood and give health education. After the intervention the spleen rates, parasite rates and fever cases dropped to nearly zero in the three study villages.

Hygiene education by female health visitors in Teknaf, Bangladesh. Communities receiving hand pumps were given health education by female health visitors over a 2-month period, through home visits, group discussions and demonstrations. An evaluation found significant improvements in hygiene practices and a reduction in diarrhoea incidence in children under 2 years in the community receiving the health education compared with other communities.

Using volunteers to reach women in Kandy, Sri Lanka. The Women's Development Centre set up a community-based programme that trained educated unemployed female volunteers. The training consisted of health education, family and child health, nutrition, communication and leadership development including legal issues. An evaluation found that, when compared with villages where the programme did not function, women in communities with functioning volunteers had a better understanding of health messages and were more likely to take their child for monthly growth monitoring and to decide for themselves about taking their sick child to see a health worker.

Peer education among sex workers in Thailand. Small groups of 5–10 sex workers received training through 2-hour sessions held every 3 months over a year. The sessions were carried out at the women's place of work and aids used included a flip chart, models of penises, and special card games and role-play games. One to three experienced women were trained as peer educators for each establishment. Influential brothel owners were selected to develop 'model brothels' to influence others in the locality. A free condom supply for sex establishments was established. Before the intervention, only 42% of women surveyed by volunteers posing as clients refused to have sex without a condom. After the peer education programme the proportion refusing increased to more than 90%.

Peer education in prisons in Mozambique. Prisoners with primary school education were selected and given 20 hours of training. Peer educators then trained other prisoners about AIDS and STDs over three educational sessions lasting 30 minutes each. Peer education was reinforced by a drama prepared by a group of prisoners. An evaluation showed that knowledge among prisoners increased especially among prisoners with less education.

Outreach to sex workers in Bali, Indonesia. Outreach workers ran educational sessions for sex workers and pimps that covered knowledge or AIDS and STDs, condoms and negotiating skills. This was supplemented by visits to their places of work to provide informal advice, hand out posters and pamphlets targeted at clients and distribute condoms, which could then be sold to clients at a profit. An evaluation found an increase in use of condoms in brothels where the education was carried out compared with others with no education.

Peer education among truck drivers in Tanzania. Female bar and guest house workers and male petrol station workers at truck stops were trained as peer educators and given ongoing support. Social welfare and transport officers at transport companies were also trained as peer educators. Health education from peer educators to drivers was reinforced with posters, stickers, pamphlets, booklets, flip charts, audiocassettes, dramas and video shows. A survey before and 18 months afterwards showed an increase in self-reported condom use by truck drivers.

or immunisation you may find that these are not the most important issues to the community. In that case you should try to involve other health workers in the initial activities.

Initial briefings

It is important that everyone involved in implementing the programme meets and carefully considers all the implications of a community participation strategy. Outside professionals such as engineers and planners may see themselves as the experts and not recognise that the community should have a say in their affairs. The health workers in the community may feel threatened by allowing people in the community to make decisions. Everyone involved should be made aware of the advantages of letting communities decide for themselves what their priorities should be.

Timescale for community participation

Another serious problem comes from the short timescale of many projects. It is not enough to make a single visit to a community and expect that everyone will join and work together. You have seen that community participation is a *process* that takes time to develop. Unfortunately many health programmes are planned on a short timescale. A 'project cycle' of 2 or 3 years is common. At the end of this period sponsors are often demanding 'results' such as completed latrines or decreases in morbidity. However, it is extremely difficult to develop genuine community participation in such a short time. Although lip-service may be paid to community participation, projects often dispense with that in the rush to meet targets.

Open-ended community oriented objectives

When setting objectives for your programmes, it is important not to be too rigid on your desired outcomes. If you are genuinely promoting community participation your objectives will be determined by the community themselves. This must be pointed out to any donor agencies who should not try to impose objectives on the community. Keep your objectives open-ended.

As the main point of community participation is to develop self-reliance, critical awareness and problem-solving skills in communities, this should be reflected in the objectives. Look at the two sets of objectives below. What differences can you see in them?

1 By the end of the programme 20 pit latrines will have been dug.
2 By the end of the programme the community would have come together to consider how they might work together to improve their community and have started on a topic of their own choice.

The first objective is based on changes in a specific health behaviour. The second objective is concerned with changes *in people* rather than

particular behaviours. These 'process' objectives deal with more fundamental changes such as self-awareness, self-empowerment and problem-solving skills.

Evaluation of community participation programmes

Evaluation involves showing that the objectives have been achieved in the most efficient manner possible. Evaluation of community participation programmes should be based, not only on achievement of specific health and behaviour changes, but also achievement of the 'process objectives' described above.

If you take community participation seriously, the community should be involved in the evaluation of the programme as well. Evaluation becomes a learning experience in which everybody looks at what has been achieved and decides what more needs to be done. There is growing interest in *participatory evaluation* and *action-research* that are described further in the final chapter of this book.

In practice, evaluation has to fulfil several distinct needs. You may be mainly concerned with looking at achievements, the effective-

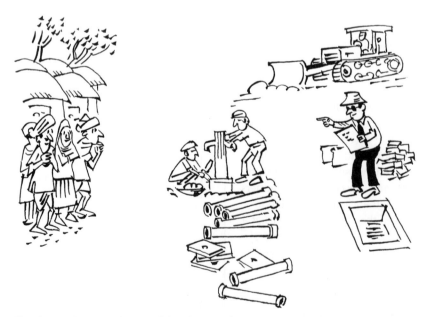

Fig. 6.11 Community participation is often ignored in the rush to get the job done

ness of your methods and whether the community has found it worthwhile. However, your employers may not understand – or be sympathetic to – the full implications of community participation and may not accept the value of outcomes that the community feels are important.

It is a good idea to include a range of indicators in the evaluation schedule that take into account both the community's as well as other key groups' interests. You can compare changes in your target community with 'control' communities where the programme is not operating. A good programme will respond to the community's needs with a flexible evaluation that adjusts to changing situations.

Need for community-based field organisers

Your community may already be united with a clear idea of its needs and an organised structure with which you can work. Then your task is an easy one. However, the initial situation is often a community divided in its interests and felt needs and poorly organised to take advantage of available resources. In that case, establishing dialogue, bringing people together, discussing felt needs and resolving conflicts will require time, effort and skill. You will need to decide who will carry out these demanding tasks. If you cannot do this yourself, you will have to involve others.

One approach is to obtain the funds to employ a special group of workers. However, while it is helpful to have full-time community workers, community participation should not be seen as something that can only be done when a programme has full-time community workers on its staff. It should be possible to train health and other field workers and adjust work schedules so that community organisation activities are built into their normal workload. Yet most health workers based in clinics and health centres receive little training on methods for working with communities.

Whoever you use to be your community organisers, they must be properly selected and trained to enable them to carry out their task effectively. Their training should enable them to: understand community structures; identify opinion leaders; be good listeners and communicators; work with individuals and groups; advise on community organisation; and use participatory learning methods.

Summary – conditions for successful community participation programmes

The most important resources for the promotion of health are the people themselves. Through community participation you can use that resource to improve the health of the people. However, it would be wrong to claim that community participation can overcome all the problems facing communities. Some health educators have been criticised for emphasising community participation while ignoring action to deal with international forces, government policies, natural disasters, poverty and exploitation. These can only be tackled at national and international level. Effective health education cannot ignore politics.

Community participation is not always a feasible strategy. You may not have the time yourself or have access to other fieldworkers for the demanding task of working with local communities, holding dialogue or supporting community organisations. Then you may have no other choice but to use approaches such as radio. In urban areas, your target group may be scattered throughout the city so it is not feasible to bring them together for common action and an outreach approach may be best. In cases of emergencies, such as an epidemic, there simply may not be the time for going through the process of community participation.

However, in most situations a genuine community participation approach is both desirable and feasible – *but can only be achieved if you plan for it*. This involves considering the problems and solutions that have been discussed in this chapter and are summarised below.

- Brief all staff on community participation.
- Involve all the relevant agencies.

- Base the programme on an understanding of the local community and their felt needs.
- Have open-ended objectives.
- Have a realistic timescale.
- Allow genuine community control.
- Use well-trained fieldworkers.

- Provide support and training for volunteer lay workers.
- Build in dialogue and participatory learning experiences.
- Involve the community in evaluation.

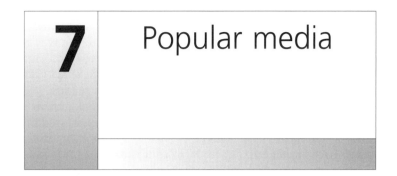

7   Popular media

Long before the coming of mass media, great religions and social ideas spread to millions of people by word of mouth. Many communities, even today, learn from, trust and enjoy the spoken word and visual image. In this chapter I will:

1 Look at a range of 'folk' or 'popular' media and consider their potential for communicating health.
2 Consider what needs to be considered in mobilising popular media for health education and health promotion.

What are popular media?

Traditional media that appear on special occasions and are only watched by a minority are an important part of a nation's history. But they are not really popular media in the sense that I will deal with in this chapter. The most important characteristic of popular media is that they are enjoyed *today*. They are *living* traditions, enjoyed by many people. Their popularity comes from:

• their entertainment value;
• their coverage of ideas and issues of universal concern such as love, marriage, honour, failure, success, jealousy, revenge, wealth, poverty, power, family and group conflicts and religion;
• the fact that even though they are based on tradition, they change and adapt with the

time to deal with new situations and incorporate the issues and concerns of the day.

Before dealing with different forms of folk media in more detail, let us consider some examples of different popular media.

• The *Calypso* is a type of song that has become highly popular in the Caribbean both through live performances, radio broadcasts and on records. The music has a fast popular beat and contains words that comment on current issues. They often criticise government actions and make fun of national institutions.
• The *Ramlilas* in India take place every year in many villages. Members of the community participate in acting out scenes from the Ramayana, the Hindu epic poem that describes the life of Rama and his battle with evil in the form of the demon king Ravana. The performances, often in the open air, involve the whole community.
• *Ngonjera* is a form of written and spoken poetry in the local Kiswahili language that became popular in Tanzania. Two or three actors act out the poem, which is often about political or social events. Media such as charts, photographs and real objects are often incorporated. Poetry is so popular that many Kiswahili newspapers reserve a page for readers' poems.
• Among the Tiv people in Nigeria a new style of theatre *Kwagh-hir* evolved combining traditional and ritual elements with a storyteller,

acrobats, dancers, puppet shows, stories and tales. In open-air performances, themes dealing with traditionalism and modernisation are performed. The Tiv people also use singing, dancing, music, drama and storytelling in their rituals, feasts and leisure activities to express their traditions. For many years the drumbeats of 'talking drums' were used to communicate over hundreds of miles and many people today still understand this language. In their music, the rhythms of the drumbeats can communicate messages to the audience.

- In the state of Kerala in Southern India trucks are elaborately decorated with **folk paintings** and **proverbs**. The decorations vary from elaborate and intricate flower designs to characters from western cartoons.
- The **merolicos** in Mexico are medicine men who set up stalls at markets and other public places and use ventriloquism, mind-reading, snake-handling and other arts to sell some medicinal products. They are treated with respect by the community. The medicine men communicate information about health in their performance.
- In West African towns and villages importance announcements are traditionally made by a **town crier**.

Folk media that have been used in health education include:

- **storytelling**   oral
             written
- **drama**   theatre as performance
             participatory theatre
             puppets
- **song**   'pop' songs
             folk song types
- **pictures**   'art'
             cloth designs

Storytelling

Storytelling is a good way to communicate health.

- Stories build on the impact of the spoken word – which is always more powerful that the written word.

- Everyone is interested in stories, they can identify themselves with the characters.
- While educated people have been trained to think in logical organised way, the story format is closer to the way most people think.
- People remember information better when it is presented in a story format rather than a formal talk or lecture.
- Stories can make truth concrete – abstract ideas can be expressed in everyday terms.
- Stories begin from the things that people understand.
- Stories can allow people to discover principles for themselves.

The health topic might form the main story. Another approach is to have the main story dealing with other topics that have a high universal appeal. These might be intrigues, quarrels, sexual liaisons, arguments, encounters with ghosts or magic and include health issues as a sub-theme.

A well-developed story will provoke a good response if people see it to be relevant to their lives. It should be told in an interesting way, changing one's voice to suit the different characters. The audience should be involved along the way with questions such as, 'Now what do you think happened next?' If people believe in the story and identify themselves with the characters they are more likely to remember the message and take action to change their situation and adopt health-promoting behaviours.

David Hilton describes how the Ladin Gabas Rural Health Programme in Nigeria used the following approach to train village health workers with stories:

1 The teacher tells the story to the class from memory then asks the class questions afterwards to see what they have learned.
2 One student is chosen to repeat the story aloud and the teacher and other students comment.
3 The class then divides into groups of four or five, each of whom then tells the story to those in his group until all have had a chance.
4 Each group then creates a drama from the stories with the students in the group each acting a part.

5. The class comes together and each group presents its drama, which is then discussed.
6. The class evaluates the performance of each group and if desired chooses the best.

Drama and popular theatre

Drama (sometimes called 'popular theatre') can also be used to promote community participation. It is a powerful way of carrying out Paulo Freire's approach to education that was described in the previous chapter.

In one approach, a drama group visits a community and develops the drama from local issues. Following presentation of the drama the community is involved in discussion issues and suggesting solutions. It is possible to stop the drama at different stages and ask for comments, suggestions or for the community to take part. You do not need professional actors and can develop a performance entirely using local community members where the process of development of the drama becomes as important as the actual performance.

A well-known example of the use of drama in this participatory way is the Laedza Batanani theatre project in Botswana. The name means in the local language 'The sun is already up – it is time to come and work together'. Its purpose was to present issues through an entertainment medium and 'wake people up' to take collective action to deal with them. They identify three stages in their approach to using drama: identification, drama scripting and performance.

In the problem *identification* stage the field workers held workshops where a committee of elders in the community was selected and between 60 to 100 community members were invited. Small group 'brainstorming' sessions were held (see Chapter 5). These produced a list of ideas from the community which could be grouped into five major categories: village development problems; family problems; value conflicts and social problems; economic concerns; and consumer concerns. The members of the community were asked to put the problems in order of importance and improvise short sketches to illustrate them.

The next stage, *drama scripting*, involved working with the persons selected by the village committee to be the actors. The actors developed the script from the ideas that had been generated earlier. They added a set of characters,

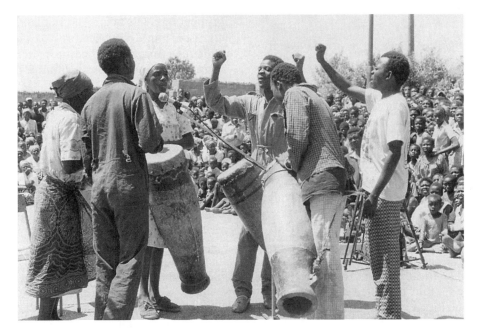

Fig. 7.1   Theatre group in Zambia

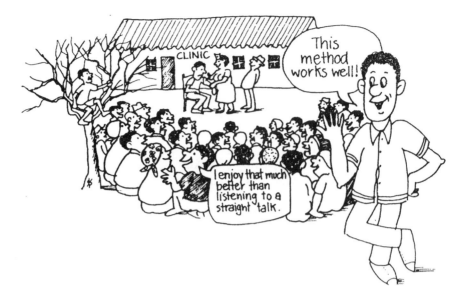

Fig. 7.2   Theatre for development in Botswana

such as a miner, a drunkard, or a grandmother, to produce a script that was entertaining but still contained key development messages.

The final stage of *performance* took place in villages and at festivals. Following each performance the actors asked the audiences to join them in small group discussion and posed the questions:

Are the problems shown in the drama real problems in your village?
How can these problems be solved?
Does the theatre project help you to overcome the problems?

Their performances also included music and dancing. Simple books were produced based on the stories in the drama and these were given out to audiences and schools. Videotapes were made of performances and these were also found to stimulate discussion.

The Liwonde Primary Health Care Unit in Malawi provides a good example of how drama can be used as part of a primary health care programme. Their theatre team visited the Mwima community to find out their problems. Their grievances included: absence of a nurse/clinical officer; lack of good protected water; lack of a proper market; existence of various diseases

such as diarrhoea, measles and scabies; and hospitals too far away.

After analysing their research findings, the team prepared a drama sketch about the location of wells in the village. The play was performed in the village *bwalo*, a square in front of the headman's house that is the traditional place for meetings. The actors did not use real objects but used mime and gestures to create in the audience's imagination features such as houses, goats, a well, a rubbish dump and babies' nappies.

The performance involved the community by directly addressing the audience on controversial issues. For example when the actor playing a villager complained to the other actor playing the headman about animals fouling the well, the question was put to the audience 'Is that true? Is that how the well is supposed to be kept?' The audience responded actively, arguing with the actors and each other about the factual and moral issues raised in the play. Since issues about water and wells in rural Malawian society are traditionally the responsibility of women, women were involved in the discussions. Following the drama and a repeat performance, the villagers agreed to work together to improve the well.

This success stimulated the villagers' enthusiasm for primary health care. The health project followed this up with a play about the election of village health committees and the importance of community participation in matters of health. Ten villages in the area formed village health committees which, supported by further drama sketches, actively promoted preventive measures. Topics covered included cementing of wells, chlorinating of wells, promotion of pit latrines and provision of basic medicines such as chloroquine, aspirin and antibiotic eye-ointment.

The success of the theatre programme in these villages led to the use of theatre in other communities. The Primary Health Care Unit held a 5-day workshop to train others village health committee members in other communities on the use of theatre for primary health care. This led to an expansion of theatre activities. An evaluation of the theatre programme was carried out in the two areas where extensive use had been made of theatre methods. Over two years, there had been an increase in latrines built and a reduction in diarrhoea. But there had been little change in a similar area where there had been no drama activities.

Mime is a form of theatre acted out without words. This is of special value when there are many languages in a community. The Jagran theatre company in India has worked in Delhi's slum colonies performing to audiences of up to 2000 people. With 14 languages and many hundred dialects, spoken theatre is almost impossible in these colonies but the language of mime communicates to all on the street or a village immediately.

Jagran have described their approach as follows:

The Jagran troupe performs in the midst of slums and villages in various states of India. It is an informal affair. The message goes round by word of mouth. And it is a matter of minutes for crowds to assemble around the troupe. On the surface the show is entertainment, humorous and lighthearted. The audience laugh at themselves. They laugh at the drunkard, at the villain who insists on dowry, at the fellow who eats dirty food and suffers from diarrhoea. But beneath the slapstick and comedy are messages aimed to make the audience view their lives in a different perspective. The actors are members of the audience, dressed like them; but for the grease paint, the comic situations are theirs and so are the tragedies. And with all this identification, communication becomes almost complete.

One of Jagran's plays is called *The monster of malnutrition*. The father and son are scared by a huge monster. They discover that this is because of their eating habits, so they change their diet to a healthy balanced one and are able to kill off the monster. The facts of nutrition are introduced in a comic humorous way so the audience are entertained but do not forget the point.

Puppets

Puppets are a form of drama with considerable potential for health education. Puppets may be part of the tradition of a country such as the Punch and Judy shown in Britain and the shadow puppets of Indonesia. One advantage of puppets is that it is possible for them to say things on sensitive topics that it would be unacceptable for an actor to say in a drama. People will accept puppets criticising traditions and institutions. So puppets are particularly valuable for dealing with controversial topics such as sex education and AIDS. In the USA they have been used to reduce the fear and anxiety that children have about going to stay in hospital or visiting the dentist.

- Different types of puppets are: *glove puppets* with heads made from paper mâché or clay; *rod puppets* with figures on wooden rods; *paper bag puppets* with faces drawn on paper bags; *jointed puppets* moved by string; and *shadow puppets* where a cardboard cutout casts a large shadow against a wall.
- Don't just wave the puppets around – make them do things – chase, nod, fight, hit, and even kiss! Practise the movements in front of a mirror – or ask people to watch and give advice on your performance.
- Give the puppets names, special clothing and personalities. Lighten the tension by including humour. Include music and songs. Keep

it simple – do not try to cover too much. Entertain – avoid preaching.

- You can make a proper stage that can be easily put up and taken down again for transportation. However, a wall or curtain for the puppeteers to stand behind is usually enough. A large piece of cloth can be hung across two trees or across a doorway or the window of a house.

- Choose the timing of performances carefully. Find out when your audience – women, children or men – are free. Choose suitable locations. Markets, festivals, agricultural shows, health committee meetings or schools all provide good opportunities to use puppets. Make sure performances are well publicised in advance.

Many people see puppets as relevant only for children and are surprised when they realise how useful they can be with adults. For example, in the Laedza Batanani theatre project in Botswana, a puppet show was given to entertain the children on the mornings of the theatre performances and the adults were also interested. The found that controversial village persons, such as the traditional healer, could be portrayed without giving offence, by using puppets.

As with drama, puppets have most impact when the community participate in the preparation of the programme, performing the show and can discuss it afterwards. Even so, puppets

can be filmed and broadcast on television and provide entertaining and interesting health education to large audiences. The American programme *Sesame Street* uses a format of real actors, puppets and songs to provide a valuable educational experience and has been watched by millions of pre-school children throughout the world.

Songs

The words and music of songs can have a powerful effect on the emotions. Musicians carry great influence and are admired and looked up to. Songs can be used to rouse people to action and good examples of this are the stirring freedom songs of the black people of South Africa and the Civil Rights protest movement in the United States. People can be heard in the streets singing the jingles from television and radio advertising.

The calypso songs of the Caribbean were one of the examples of popular media that I gave you at the beginning of this chapter. The calypso below was sung and composed in the local English dialect by 'The Mighty Sheller', who was a leading calypso singer in the island of St Vincent.

They say ninety thousand, is our population.
One hundred and fifty square miles of land,

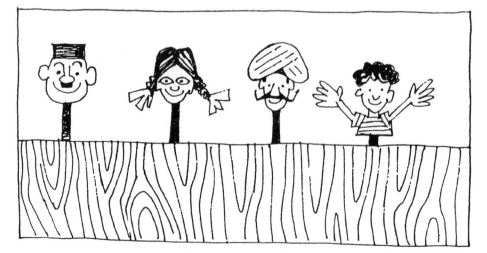

Fig. 7.3   Puppets

For we to live on.
One fifth of the population is strong and
  healthy women.
Don't doubt everyone of them could produce
  children.

Chorus: There is a need I see, in this country.
  So start plan your family.
  Otherwise is more delinquency.
  More crime and poverty.
  So do some family planning, and
    help the situation.
  Join St Vincent Planned Parenthood
    Association.

Young men of this country I want you to
  realise.
If you join in this exercise, you can get yourself sterilise.
Come take the operation, it is simple and
  quite easy.
That wouldn't prevent you from enjoying
  sexual activity.

Our local association will give you some good
  advice.
When you need it come and visit, the staff is
  helpful and nice.
So my fellow Vincentian, I am telling you in
  advance.
I feel family planning is of national importance.

The Ladin Gabas project in Nigeria that was
described earlier in the chapter also uses songs.
The song leader sings the story, while the others
join in the chorus after each verse. The song
below is one they developed to tell about the
symptoms, cause, prevention and treatment of
malaria.

Chorus: Good health we want
  Let's all be healthy.

Verses: Fever is bothering me,
  Mosquitoes bring it.
  Standing water around out house
  causes mosquitoes to breed.
  Let us take the children to the clinic.
  That they may stay well.
  We take them to the clinic for
  Daraprim.
  That they may stay well.

Broken pots and tin pans.
Let us bury them.

In a nutrition project in Uganda, a popular
ballad singer was asked to compose a song about
kwashiorkor and its prevention. The song he
prepared, called *'Kitobero'*, was made available
as a record and was a great success. Songs have
been used in education of the public on AIDS in
many countries and are particularly valuable in
reaching young people. One project in Zaire
recorded songs about AIDS and installed cassette
recorders on public buses to play the songs to
the passengers.

Songs were also an important part of the
health education programme directed at the
young people aged 13–18 years in 11 countries including Mexico, Peru and Bolivia. The
message 'It's OK to say no' was the theme of
the campaign that was directed at reducing
the incidence of teenage pregnancies. Following initial research, it was found that the most
important interest of the young people was
music and the project produced two songs,
one on each side of a record, with a colour
record jacket which opened into an attractive
poster.

Focus group discussions (see Chapter 11 for
more detail on this research method) were carried out. These established the acceptability of
the following points: (1) young people, both
men and women, should be sexually responsible
for their own actions; (2) it's OK to say no; (3)
young people can go to specific identified places
for professional counselling or guidance; and 4)
positive role models, i.e. persons they look up
to, are helpful to young people who want to be
responsible.

The singers were carefully chosen to appeal
to the young people and who accepted the main
messages in their own lives. Tatiana, a young
Mexican woman and Johnny a young Puerto
Rican man were selected. A competition was
held with more than 20 professional composers
participating to select five songs. The final
choice of two, selected by pre-testing with
groups of young people, were: 'When we are
together' and 'Wait'. These were marketed as
commercial songs with the usual promotional
material to accompany them.

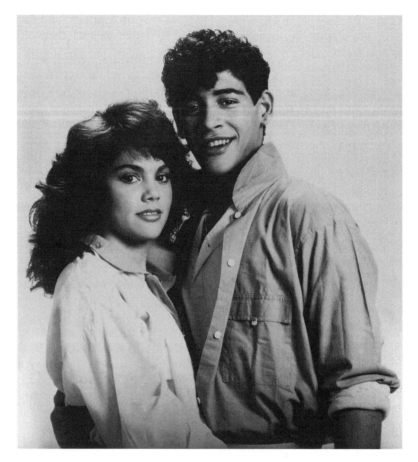

Fig. 7.4   Tatiana and Johnny

The words for one of their songs were:

> *She:*   There's no need to run, there is
> no need to run.
> Love that is rushed, is love that is
> lost.
> *Chorus:*   Understand!
> *Both:*   Let's not love at the wrong time.
> *Chorus:*   Stop!

The songs reached top of the hit parade in Mexico within 6 weeks of their release. Not only were the songs heard by millions of young people, but they even made a profit that could be spent on further projects for young people. Patrick Coleman, from the Population Communication Services of Johns Hopkins University who managed this exciting and innovative programme, draws the following lessons from their experience:

- Choose the most appropriate medium to reach the intended audience, in this case popular music.
- Involve professionals who are experienced in the chosen medium and make sure they are the best available.
- Develop a high quality product that will attract the commercial sector. Commercial support for a social message helps to meet production expenses, assures wider spread of the message, and may even generate income for programme expansion.
- Use a medium, in this case popular music, that has a big regional and national audience. This enables a large-scale project to draw on resources not readily available to a local organisation working alone and brings additional attention to the project because of its international scope.

Working on this large scale needs considerable initial funding and may not be possible for you. But it should still be possible for you to use music and songs in your community. The principle of involving local musicians and maintaining a high standard of entertainment also applies – even for community-based projects.

Songs can be used to promote community participation and challenge social injustice. A programme working in the Dominican Republic started a Nutrition Education and Recuperation Centre in a poor section of the provincial capital of Barahona. Meetings were held with the women who discussed family planning and sex, prevention of disease, and the promotion of good health in low-income communities. The women made wall posters from cuttings from newspapers and magazines, they composed and learned songs and carried out some drama on a social issue. The songs they sing deal with social issues.

Let me tell you, my friend.
These days we can't cope,
Rice costs 34 cents,
And it's 40 cents for soap.

In the neglected slums,
We're tired of having to say:
Light costs too much
And we can't afford to pay.

Chorus: Onward, women, onward!
Together we must strive,
Let us unite
To better our lives

Visual art

Another form of popular media that can be used in health education is visual art. Magazines and newspapers are often dominated by 'commercial art' which is often based on western pictures. However, most cultures have traditional forms of visual art. In societies where the level of literacy is low, pictures often have a specific purpose of telling stories. Examples of this are the religious paintings and stained glass windows of early Christian Europe and temple carvings and religious wall paintings of India. These tradition-

al visual art forms show themselves in many ways; from the decorations on houses, religious buildings, temples, trucks, and public buildings; carvings in wood and stone; designs on fabrics and clothes; and posters, paintings and calendars.

In Ghana there are traditional symbols that have quite specific meanings. One symbol, 'Sankofa', means combining traditional with modern and was used as the title of a WHO film describing a primary health programme in Ghana.

In Sri Lanka the accelerated national immunisation adopted a symbol based on the traditional *pachayudhya* symbol used from ancient times to ward off evil and disease especially in children. The trident, chank, sword, bow and arrow and amulets are symbols to conquer disease and malevolent spirits.

There are many examples of the use of folk art and design in health education communication.

Other popular media

Once we start looking carefully we can uncover other forms of popular communication that could be used in health education. In many streets and markets there are street merchants selling goods, including medicines, charms and traditional ointments. There might be fortune tellers and street entertainers. Listen to them and you can learn a great deal from the methods they use to attract interest and persuade people to buy their products.

In the towns of Nepal there are fortune tellers who tell the future from cards. A health education project produced, with help from UNICEF, an additional card that contained a goddess on one side and a diagram promoting oral rehydration solution on the other.

Some problems in using popular media

Communities may see folk media as a form of entertainment and not as something that pro-

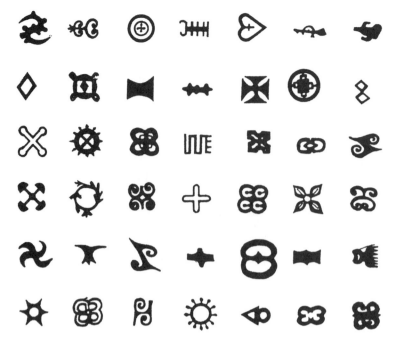

Fig. 7.5   Ghana Ashanti symbols

motes learning. There is also a risk that, in attempting to make folk media as entertaining as possible, health messages may become lost. Actors and musicians in the excitement of performance may improvise and distort health messages. An evaluation of a programme in Ghana that used songs to teach about AIDS found that people liked to dance to the music and sing the songs but did not take any notice of the messages!

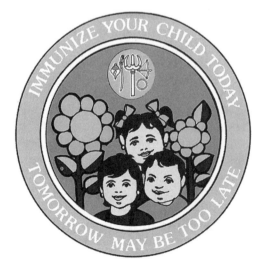

Fig. 7.6   Sri Lanka immunisation sticker with traditional 'pachayudhya' symbol

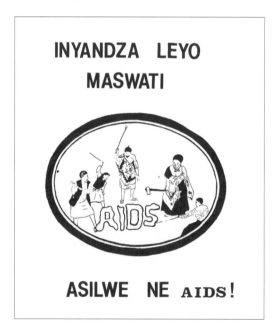

Fig. 7.7   Swaziland AIDS leaflet with traditional design

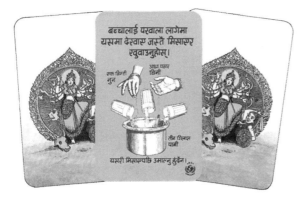

Fig. 7.8   Fortune-telling card promoting oral rehydration therapy in Nepal

While folk media can be very effective, they will only have an impact on a problem if they are seen and heard by large numbers of people, which usually means doing more than just a single performance. A great deal of organisation and expense for food, transport and salaries can be involved in taking performers around repeating performances in different communities. It is also important to make sure that there is proper advance preparation and follow-up in each setting. If the performers are health workers or members of the community, there are limits to the time they can spend on folk media. If they are professional musicians, they will expect to have a proper payment for their efforts. Careful thought is needed on making the use of folk media *sustainable* – how to *deliver* the folk media and how much this will cost.

Even a well-designed programme can easily go wrong. The Family Planning Council of Nigeria and the International Planned Parenthood Association collaborated to use the Yoruba traditional travelling theatre 'opera' form as a basis for a film for family planning motivation. A well-known and respected actor Kola Ogunmola, leader of a troupe of travelling players, was asked to participate. Ognumola was involved in production of the final script and the play was filmed in a Yoruba village with his company playing the main roles and local people as extras.

The story centred on the dilemma facing a forward-looking urban family who planned their family. They returned to their village for a wedding and saw the difficulties their brother faced in providing for his large family. The rural brother asked the town-dwelling brother to take one of his sons with him and look after him and a disagreement arose. The new bride is taken aside and instructed about the value of family planning. The film *My Brother's Children* was produced in Yoruba and English and shown widely in family planning branches, health centres, clinics and hospitals. Twenty thousand copies of a comic strip featuring the same story were also distributed. Showing of the film was followed by discussions by the health workers.

Despite all the careful preparations, the programme is generally considered to have been a failure. A detailed evaluation was undertaken by researchers at Ibadan University which identified some reasons for the film's lack of success. The evaluation showed that, although understood and enjoyed by health and family planning workers, it had less impact on the community for which it was intended. The rural audience did not have much experience of films so the novelty of the film show and projector distracted them from the content and the film, lasting almost an hour, contained too much.

The film had been pre-tested with health workers, not the community, so the content did not fit into the local culture – for example in one scene the family elder gave the bride, not only his blessing, but advice on her future role. This was seen by the audience to be inappropriate behaviour. The messages of the film mainly reflected the ideas and thought processes of the health and family planning workers rather than how the community themselves saw family planning and their needs. In fact, the character the audience identified with, and felt sympathy for, was not the progressive brother using family planning but the brother living in the village with his large family!

My Brother's Children gives us important lessons and reinforces the points made in other chapters in this book – especially understanding behaviour. The impact of popular media is stronger with a live performance compared with the same performance on film – especially if film is an unfamiliar medium. Even if you are using popular artists who are close to the culture of the community, you will need to pre-test your messages with members of the intended audience. Better still, you should involve the community in choosing the messages and ideas to put across in the drama. Perhaps the most important lesson, however, is that it is not enough to use an entertaining medium to promote change. If the ideas and practices you are trying to promote are radically different from and incompatible with what the community are now practising, and require accompanying economic and social changes, you probably won't succeed!

Production process for popular media

The production process for using popular media is shown in Figure 7.10.

Development of the content

Development of the popular media involves having discussions about what to put in it, where to do it and how to make sure that the performance is as good as possible.

The biggest challenge when using popular media is to get the right balance between health content and entertainment. If it is a drama, it is important that sufficient time is allowed to allow proper development of the characters or

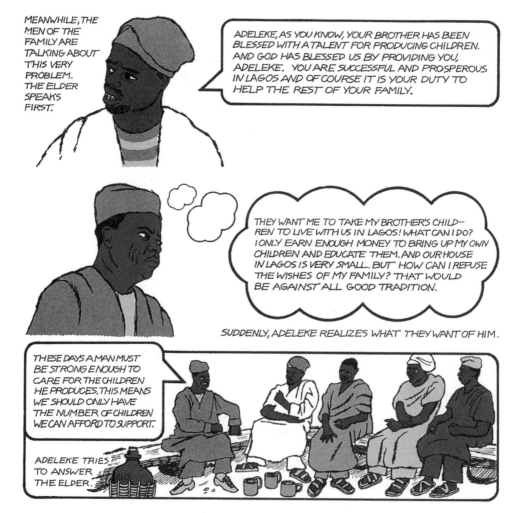

Fig. 7.9   Extract from cartoon storybook accompanying the Nigerian film *My Brother's Children*

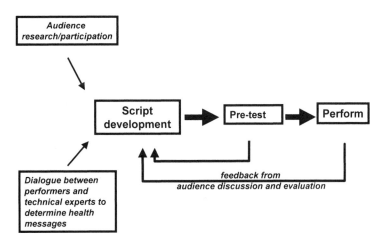

Fig. 7.10   Production process for using popular media

the plot of a story. The audience should identify with the situation and the persons portrayed. If the health message is too obvious, it can be boring and result in the audience 'turning off'. However, it is also possible that a health message can be hidden by a storyline that is entertaining but too complicated.

A critical issue is who should write the script for the plays or the music and words for the songs. It is also important to ensure that the content of the popular media takes into account community understandings and perception. This could involve drawing upon any existing research or carrying out new research. Another approach is to involve members of the target group in developing the popular media, so that their concerns and feelings are reflected. The development of the content will also need some input from health workers to identify important health messages. However, most health workers do not have expertise in popular media so care has to be taken not to put too much medical information into the content.

Traditional musicians, actors, puppeteers and artists are good communicators with an understanding of what communities find interesting and entertaining. They have skills in developing plots, music and stories that will hold an audience's interest. However, if the development of the folk media is left completely with musicians there is a risk that the performance will be entertaining but the health messages may be distorted

or lost. A *team* approach is needed – involving the community, health workers, and traditional performers to make use of all of their skills.

Programmes using folk media have used the following approaches in selection of performers:

- *Professional actors and singers.* The quality of the performance can be very high but it is important to make sure that the content is relevant to the community. Funds will have to be found for salaries.
- *Volunteers.* A group of health workers can do the drama in their spare time. This can be a useful approach but time commitments of the volunteers may limit their availability for repeat performances.
- *Members of the target community,* e.g. youth group, women's group, school children. Involvement in the process of development of a drama can have a valuable impact on the performers' own lives as well as the impact on the community who watch them. This is a good approach for reaching a particular community, but not a suitable one if the aim is to take the performance to many communities to reach a large number of people.

Another important decision is where the perform should be done. There are two options that are widely used.

- *Fixed location* – e.g. in a community hall, open meeting, outside a clinic/health centre, at a school or parents' evening. In these situations the audience is fixed and around for most of the performance, which can last up to 1 or 2 hours. There is more opportunity for dialogue and participation by the audience.

- *Public place* – in streets, markets, fairs and other open air locations. The aim is to reach people who are passing but may not stay for very long because of other commitments. Performances have to be short and include repetition so that even if you only stay for 10 minutes you will still get a message. The opportunities for questions and participation by the audience are more limited.

Pre-testing

Pre-testing the performance will ensure that the content is appropriate, is understandable and is acceptable to the intended audience. This involves bringing together a group that is representative of the intended audience. After they have seen the performance the audience can be put in groups of about eight persons and asked questions to find out their views on the performance and to check for recall, understanding, acceptability and the appropriateness of the messages.

Evaluation

Evaluation involves obtaining feedback from the audiences on the impact of the performance. This can be done by interviewing the members of the audience before and after performances. Another approach is to have focus group discussions with members of the audience after performances. This is useful to get in-depth feedback on reactions. Some of the indicators you can use include:

- *Coverage* – How many people watched/heard the folk media?
- *Short-term impact* – Immediately after the performance was there increase in knowledge, acceptance of message, lack of negative reaction?
- *Long-term impact,* e.g. after 2–3 months or even longer. Whether people still remember

the message; whether they have started to put the message into practice; whether there has been a change in behaviour; whether records of health facilities indicate changes in utilisation by community; sales of medicines by pharmacists; receipts of dumped unwanted expired medicines.

Case studies of the use of popular media for health promotion

Puppets against AIDS in South Africa. Dramas were performed by puppets 2 metres high. The company arrive at the venue, usually a busy centre. The activity begins to attract a crowd, then music and drums and announcements over a public address system attract people – and finally the puppets appear to the waiting crowd. The story describes how Joe, who is infected with HIV, passes the infection to others through sex with his girlfriends before eventually dying of AIDS. Typical audiences reached in each showing were between 100 and 500 persons. An evaluation measured the impact on the audience through an interview and questionnaire survey before and after the shows. Almost all persons interviewed said they enjoyed the show and there were improvements in knowledge.

'Ms Rumours' street theatre in urban areas of Peru. The play was performed in parks and squares and also outside hospitals and clinics to people waiting for services. Each performance lasted about 20 minutes and was followed by a group question-and-answer session. The story involved four characters, Ms Rumours, a couple in love and a pharmacist. The street theatre showed how Ms Rumours promotes misconceptions and negative attitudes, and shows the pharmacist dispelling those rumours. From April 1992 to July 1994 the play was performed about 200 times to an estimated total audience of about 61,000. About 4500 persons were motivated to attend follow-up face-to-face counselling sessions. The evaluation found the play changed knowledge but did not have an effect on attitudes.

Drama and leaflets on AIDS in west coast of Sri Lanka. A total of 58 performances were held in the evening and lasted about 2 hours. Dramas, performed by volunteers, showed the causes and consequences of HIV/AIDS. Flyers/leaflets illustrating specific facts about HIV/AIDS were given out at the dramas and at other public sites, such as bus stations. The evaluation showed increases in self-reported knowledge about HIV/AIDS and an increased awareness of personal susceptibility to HIV/AIDS.

Nalamdana theatre group in Tamil Nadu State, India produced three plays to disseminate HIV/AIDS information. An average of 1000 people attended each performance which lasted between 1 and 2 hours. A total of 121,000 people attended the dramas. Questionnaires given to audiences before and after performances suggested that the drama reduced misconceptions about AIDS and increased the levels of reported intentions to treat HIV-positive individuals more kindly.

Zuia Mbu (Kiswahili for 'prevent mosquitoes') social marketing programme for promoting insecticide-treated nets in two rural districts in south-western Tanzania. Community theatre was carried out alongside other promotional activities including posters, leaflets, billboards, songs, a raffle and speeches from community leaders. Also 37 young people were appointed in the same villages and trained as agents to sell nets and promote on-going treatment of nets with insecticides. A total of 22,410 nets and 8072 treatments were sold during the first year.

Summary

Look out for folk and popular media in your own community and see if you can mobilise them for health education. Popular media have enormous potential for health education and health promotion. In using popular media you should consider the following:

1 You can brief the artists, actors and musicians, but let them put the health topics in their own words.
2 Any health education carried out through folk media should be based on some initial research on what the community knows, feels and believes about the topic. Pre-test any folk media with a sample of the intended audience.
3 Involving communities themselves in putting together a drama can be a powerful stimulus for developing community awareness and raising consciousness. It also makes sure that the ideas presented are meaningful and relevant and are more likely to be understood and acted on.
4 You will have more impact by performing live in front of the audience especially if there is an opportunity for discussion and dialogue between actors and audience. However well-planned and properly tested, folk media can still have a valuable impact when broadcast through mass media such as film, television and radio and played on audio and videocassettes.
5 In using folk media for health avoid moralising and preaching. Don't destroy their essential characteristics: their popular nature; their entertainment value and ability to deal with social issues.
6 Evaluate the impact of your performances and be prepared to change your approach in the light of feedback from audiences.

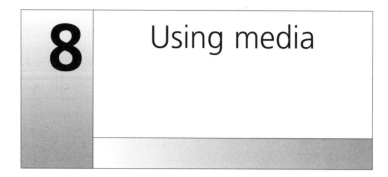

8 Using media

More and more people in the world have access to some form of mass media such as television, newspapers and radio. In Chapter 2 mass media were compared with other approaches. Mass media are often poorly used to promote one-way 'top-down' communication. However, it is possible to make effective use of media for the promotion of health by applying the guidelines described in earlier chapters, including understanding the audience, pre-testing the message and evaluating impact. This chapter will build on these earlier chapters and:

1 Look at ways in which you can use radio, television and newspapers to communicate health.
2 Give guidelines on how you can to produce your own media programmes.
3 Suggest ways of influencing the media to give publicity to your health education and health promotion work.
4 Describe ways in which you can use the media as a resource in your contacts with the community.

Media can seem expensive, difficult to use and to require special skills. Not surprisingly, many people feel powerless to use media. In this chapter I will also look at simple ways you can use the media by getting journalists to report on your activities.

The media revolution

The twenty-first century is a time of intense social change. One of the most important factors contributing to this change will be the increase in the numbers of people with some form of access to media. Many problems of visual literacy and unfamiliarity with the conventions of films, television and pictures will disappear as more and more people become exposed to different kinds of media.

Radio is the media channel that reaches the widest audience. The world is rapidly reaching a situation where most people will have access to a radio either in their family or in their community. There can be problems of distance from transmitters, poor reception in mountain terrain and supply of electricity (though the increased use and availability of wind-up radios means that batteries are not always necessary). Many countries still depend on centralised production of broadcast programmes. However, local radio stations that produce programmes in regional languages and with locally relevant content are increasingly common.

According to UNESCO there are an estimated 1400 million television receivers in the world – one for every four persons. Most of these are in the industrialised countries but the numbers are rapidly increasing in the developing countries – especially the cities, towns and nearby rural populations. In the 1980s the number of televisions in the developing countries doubled and by 1997 reached 720 million – one for every 6 persons with the highest TV ownership in Asia, Latin America and the Caribbean. The problem of the short range of television transmission is being overcome with the development of satellites.

In the industrialised countries, the expansion of television has led to a fall in the number of people going to see films in cinemas. However, the film-going audience in many developing countries is still large, especially in Asia. In some countries there has been a shift in film-going with people viewing films, not at movie houses, but on video.

Video-cassette recorders (VCR) enable audiences to view programmes, even if they are outside the range of TV broadcasts. Equipment is now widely available to project videos onto large screens so that they can be watched by many people. Some development projects have equipped mobile video units to show video programmes to rural areas.

As literacy and education increase, so does the potential of print media such as newspapers, books and magazines. More magazines are being published covering a wide range of special interests from football, music, news events, health and films.

Posters, which can range in size from quite small to large 'billboards', are another type of media used by commercial advertisers and health educators.

The most important development in media in recent years is the growth of the Internet. Anyone who is connected via a computer to the Internet has immediate access to a vast amount of information on every conceivable health topic. In developing countries the Internet is mainly used for communication with others through electronic mail (e-mail), and as a resource for health and other workers to update themselves on particular health topics. However, with the expansion of the on-line community it is only a matter of time before the Internet becomes a major force through which the public can gain access to information to improve the health and conditions in their community.

How effective are mass media?

In Chapter 3, the effectiveness of mass media was compared with face-to-face communication. Mass media messages tend to be general and they are not always relevant to the needs of individual communities. It is also difficult to be selective and to target one age group. And, unlike face-to-face approaches, there is no direct feedback. However, if used well, mass media has the great advantage of being able to reach a large audience rapidly – and does not require an infrastructure of committed fieldworkers. Although many people will prefer face-to-face communication, lack of time, the shortage of fieldworkers and difficulties of transport can make mass media the only realistic way of working.

Mass media are sometimes used poorly with a lack of audience research, dull programmes and inappropriate messages. In fact, well-planned mass media health education can achieve a great deal:

- *Behaviour change* – when the behaviour is a 'one-time' behaviour such as attending an immunisation clinic, simple to perform, or the community is favourably disposed to implement it and are merely requiring a trigger for action.
- *Agenda setting* – bringing an issue to the public's attention so that they begin talking about it and raising it at meetings.
- *Creating a favourable climate of knowledge and opinion* – media can provide specific knowledge about issues that will influence felt needs of communities; they can provide a favourable background for community-based programmes and health education activities at clinics.
- *Telling people about new ideas* – media can make people aware of new discoveries or 'innovations' such as oral rehydration. Whether people will actually act on this information depends on the idea, its complexity and whether it meets a perceived need in the community.

Who uses media?

You have already seen that, in order for a communication to be effective, it must be specific for the intended audience. Different media reach different groups in the community: people who are not literate will not read newspapers; television may only be watched by people in towns – and only those who have the money to afford it; and programmes broadcast in the daytime will not reach those at work.

So it is important to find out if your intended audience watches television, listens to the radio or reads newspapers or magazines. If they do, find out *when* they watch and *which* programmes they like. This information may already be available. It is common for newspapers, radio and television stations to carry out research on the size and characteristics of their audiences and readers. Try to find out if audience surveys have been carried out and if the results are available.

Audience surveys may not be available, so look for opportunities to find out which media your intended audience uses and likes. An example of this was the AIDS Control Programme in Swaziland which carried out a survey of youth to find out which radio programmes young people listened to. This information was used to design radio programmes that would reach as many young people as possible.

Decisions on advice to be presented on media

The concepts introduced in earlier chapters on the influences on health, understanding behaviour and communication all need to be taken into account when considering what information to include in media. As you can see in Figure 3.6, advice should be epidemiologically correct, realistic, acceptable and easy to understand. As you do not have the chance to obtain direct feedback from an audience you should always carefully pre-test the message, words, pictures and ideas to make sure that they are clear, relevant and acceptable.

Choice of formats

In the past, formats used by health educators have been mainly advertisements, spot announcements and health talks. The public can regard advertisements as a nuisance that interrupts favourite programmes. It can be a time for leaving the room to go to the toilet or putting on the kettle for a cup of tea! Many people develop resistance to the obvious sales pressure of commercial advertising and persuasive messages used in health education. However, there are many other ways to present information on health in ways that are both entertaining and effective. Success has been achieved using interviews, dramas, popular music, and stories that use traditional and cultural forms. I have listed some of these different formats below. An outline of a typical magazine format is given on page 146. Which formats do you think might be the best ones for communicating your health messages?

Social marketing – can health be sold as a product?

Social marketing is the name given to the approach of applying commercial advertising methods to promoting healthy behaviours. Social marketers place emphasis on the 'four P's': product, price, place and promotion.

- *Product* – the suggested action/behaviour change must be relevant, necessary and presented in an attractive way.
- *Price* – the product must be affordable.
- *Place* – the product must be accessible and available where the people are.
- *Promotion* – effort must be put into telling people about the product, repeating key messages in an attractive way.

The social marketing approach has been used to promote oral rehydration solution (ORS), condoms and mosquito nets. In each case, attention was paid to design of packaging and giving suitable names to make the products attractive and interesting. Care was also taken to stock local shops with them at affordable prices. They were

Formats in newspapers and magazines

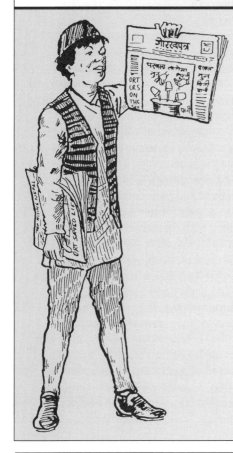

News. Descriptions of recent events often accompanied by photographs.

Future events. Details of future events, public announcements.

Advertisements. These can be any size from 'small ads' up to full page advertising commercial products and even contain health messages.

Features. Features are longer articles describing events, reviewing topics. They do not necessarily deal with news events and can contain items of general interest, short stories, science topics, advice for readers on finance. Health is often a subject for features such as descriptions of a new disease or problems of rural communities, etc.

Letters. These are usually sections with letters from the public responding to issues in previous editions of the newspaper or topics of current interest. The letters section is always popular so it is a good idea to send in your letters on health topics.

Special interest sections, including: women's page, food section, finance, sports page. Often these contain an 'advice column' responding to issues raised by readers, which can include health or even relationships with other persons.

Formats on radio and television

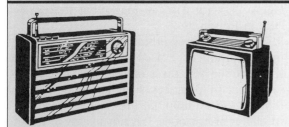

News. On most radio and television stations news bulletins are an important part of the daily output. If it is a local radio station, local news will also be included. To have your health education activity mentioned in a news bulletin is highly desirable because it gives it widespread coverage, credibility, importance and does not cost you anything.

Spot announcements. These can be public service announcements such as clinic opening times, immunisation sessions and availability of counselling services. These will usually be broadcast free. On commercial stations it is also possible to 'buy time' in the form of commercials. This could be useful for a campaign.

Slogans and jingles. Slogans are catchy short sentences, designed to attract attention, usually based on well-known sayings or rhymes. They can identify a campaign. Jingles are slogans set to music and can make a slogan more memorable, be used to identify a programme, person, radio station or theme.

Discussions. There are many kinds of discussion programmes. The one most commonly used on radio is the 'group' or 'round-table' discussion. A group of people of different opinions and from possible different backgrounds discuss a common subject under the guidance of a chairperson.

'Phone-in' programmes. A programme in which listeners ring in to the studio either 'live' or 'off-air' and give their views, ask questions or ask for advice. Their calls are dealt with either by the broadcaster, or by an expert in the studio, or by a panel involved in discussion.

Interviews. A discussion in question-and-answer form between the broadcaster and one (or two) guests. The interview can also be used to find out opinions of the 'man in the street' either in a studio situation or outside in the community (when it is then called 'vox pop').

Talks and documentaries. Five-to-fifteen minute talks by one person are occasionally used but, unless the broadcaster is very skilled, can be boring. Documentaries explore a single topic and include different effects, e.g. drama, music, interview, storytelling, descriptions, sound effects.

Drama. Long or short plays, 'soap opera', comedy sketches, serials, drama/documentaries. 'Soap opera' is the name for a weekly or even daily drama series using the same characters such as the South African soap opera *Soul City*. As discussed in Chapter 7, drama has enormous potential for health education because the audience can identify with the characters and their problems. Soap operas are even more powerful because the characters can become like family friends.

Music. This is an essential part of broadcasting, whether it is traditional music, or popular local music, musical jingles or background music to programmes. Music will attract people to watch and listen, and 'spot' announcements, public service messages and slogans can be inserted in music programmes. Jingles or songs with a message can become very popular and people will sing them and remember the message.

Quizzes and panel games. Quizzes with panels of guests are popular and most people watching or listening try to answer the questions themselves and learn something from the answers. It is a good idea to ask the listeners/viewers to write in with the correct answer to a question, and to give a prize. This gives feedback on how many people heard the programme and understood the message.

Magazine programmes. This popular format combines different short elements: music, drama, stories, sketches, interviews, comedy and discussion. The elements are linked by a presenter and are sometimes aimed at a particular audience such as women, farmers or young people. An example of a typical magazine programme is given below.

Example of typical 30-minute magazine programme and how it could be used in social development

Music:	Theme music
Announcer:	Introduction and highlights
	Music
	Soap opera episode or drama
	Music
Announcer:	Link with announcement about theme of programme
	Story or interview or local feature
	Talk by expert related to theme, or by announcer
	Music
Announcer:	Quiz related to theme of programme
	Music
Announcer:	Answers and conclusion
	Theme music

promoted with songs, jingles, posters and eye-catching campaign symbols called 'logos'. See Figure 3.14 for a social marketing strategy for ORS in Honduras.

Can the same methods for promoting commercial products be used to promote health? It is easy to see how these methods can be used for some health practices such as condoms, oral rehydration solution, latrines, vehicle seat belts, special weaning foods. It is not so easy to see the method applied to other health behaviours, such as keeping to one faithful partner or spacing one's children.

But, even if we can't apply commercial advertising on the scale of large companies, there are important lessons that we can apply: researching the target audiences, ensuring the desired practice is relevant, affordable and easy to carry out; making sure that programmes are attractive, well-presented and pre-tested; being

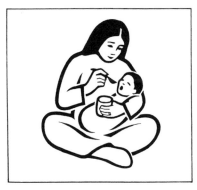

Fig. 8.1 This logo, used on Egyptian packets of oral rehydration salts, was adopted after pre-testing with groups of women in the community

aware of the importance of evaluating the impact and using the results of evaluations for future planning.

Influencing the media

You may not be in a position to prepare radio or television programmes, and feel that much of what is described above is not relevant to your situation. However, making your own programmes is only one of many different ways of using media. Indeed, it can be easier, cheaper and more effective to encourage newspapers, radio and television to take up health issues in their general news and programme content.

It is worthwhile finding out the names of the journalists and writers who put together programmes on the television and radio and write for local newspapers and magazines. They will usually be looking out for interesting stories. You can meet informally and tell them about some of the health issues you are involved in and:

- suggest some health topics that could be included in a drama they are preparing – for example one of the characters might develop a health problem and receive advice from another person;
- provide background papers on health topics and copies of any leaflets – make yourself available if they need someone to interview;

- provide questions on health topics that could be included in a quiz programme;
- write letters responding to topics covered in the newspaper or current affairs that they can put in their letters page.

You may feel that what you are doing is worthwhile and important. However, in order for it to receive coverage by the media two conditions will have to be fulfilled: *your activity has to be something that the media will see as 'newsworthy'*; and *you have to tell the media what is happening*.

Newspapers, television and radio are always looking out for something interesting to report. They keep a diary of local events and decide which are sufficiently interesting to make it worth sending a reporter to cover the event. But they are usually very busy so will only be attracted if the topic is:

- of *interest* to the community – a programme to deal with a serious disease, a visit by a famous person, activities by local community leaders;
- *topical* and relevant to other issues in the news;
- *unusual*, strange;
- anything *new* such as the launching of a new campaign; or
- a *scandal* or controversial topics such as commercial companies promoting dangerous products.

You should look out for activities in your health education programmes that might be of interest to the media. You can even deliberately include 'media events' into your programme to attract the press. Some examples of what can be done are: a ceremony with invited guests to launch a new campaign; a celebration with invited guests to mark an anniversary – the first year of the immunisation programme, the hundredth latrine to be completed, the thousandth child to receive measles immunisation; an exhibition with an official opening ceremony; an announcement of a 'new discovery'; and a presentation of prizes for a competition.

Look for opportunities for making your media events even more interesting. One approach is to invite well-known people as guests. For example, in Lesotho the Ministry of Health invited their King to launch their immunisation programme and be photographed giving oral polio vaccine to a baby.

You should also look for ways of making it *visually interesting* so that newspapers will want to include a photograph. People can be dressed in costumes, a procession carrying a coffin with the number of children who have died of the disease, a latrine can be carried on the back of a truck through the town.

As part of your media event, you could set up a *press conference* which is a meeting where journalists can ask questions and find out information. It is always a good idea to put important information on a sheet of paper as reporters can easily make mistakes in reporting technical information. The best way to let the media know what you are doing by preparing a *'Press release'* (see Figure 8.2). This is a written document of not more than one page in length, neatly typed with an attention-getting headline. It should provide information on what you are doing by answering these questions:

- *WHAT will be happening?* Describe the event. Give names of important people participating and details of activities that might make a good photograph.
- *WHY will it take place?* Give background details; explain why the activity is taking place. Supply some facts and figures that they can quote in a story – e.g. how many children died of pneumonia last year in that community.
- *WHERE will it take place?* Give precise details of how to get there.
- *WHEN will it take place?* Give the date and time of day.

In addition to background information on the topic the press release should also give an address and telephone number of someone to contact if they need further information.

WORLD AIDS DAY SPECTACULAR

On December 1st, World AIDS Day, a procession of floats and marching bands will begin at the City Hall at 10 a.m. and proceed through Main Street to City Square. They will then be addressed by a group of community leaders including the Mayor, the Chief Medical Officer, the captain of the national football team, the Minister for Woman's Affairs and the Archbishop. The highlight of the festival will be the release of 8000 balloons, one for each person who has died of AIDS this year. That night at 8 p.m. a candle-light vigil will be held at the Cathedral and Grand Mosque.

Background information: 8000 people have died of AIDS in our country so far. Surveys have shown that between 5 and 10 per cent of the public are carriers of the AIDS virus – healthy but capable of infecting others. Already 200 babies have died of AIDS this year. There is no vaccine for AIDS. Treatment is difficult and not completely effective. So the emphasis must be on prevention. Everyone should be encouraged to:

- keep to one regular sexual partner;
- avoid having sex with others whom you suspect have multiple partners or go to sex workers;
- when in doubt about your sexual partner use a condom during intercourse;
- report to your nearest clinic for treatment if you think you have a sexually transmitted disease.

For further information:
James Munyango, Coordinator World AIDS Day Celebrations tel. 54380
Joy Kalemaro, Publicity coordinator, AIDS Forum tel. 54620

Fig. 8.2   A sample press release

Before you issue the press release there are some points to consider: are you allowed by your employers to contact the press and make statements to press or radio? Will you need clearance? If you are not allowed, is there someone who can be asked to speak on your behalf? Are you sure that the information you are providing is both technically correct and fits in with national policy?

It is likely that a reporter will want to interview you for further information. You might be asked to give an interview on radio or television. This will give a valuable opportunity to get key points across but you must be well prepared! Discuss in advance the questions that will be asked. Do not be afraid to suggest additional questions the interviewer may not have thought of. Some tips to help you give an effective interview are presented below.

Tips for being interviewed on radio and television

1. Be prepared – know your facts and figures or have details handy.
2. Be clear and concise; keep to the point. If time is limited make sure that you get the most important points across first; why it is important, who is affected and what people can do about it.
3. Make it interesting! Sound enthusiastic. Have notes to refer to but try to avoid reading them out, as this will sound boring. Build in personal examples, human stories (but be careful of giving names and breaching confidentiality).
4. Keep the language simple and avoid technical words. Give statistics in ways people will easily grasp (rather than saying 15% of children die in the first year, try saying 'one in six children die' or 'every hour a baby dies of malnutrition').
5. Make it clear when you are speaking on behalf of an organisation and when you are giving your own views.
6. Keep calm! If you don't like a question, don't refuse to answer but take a lesson from politicians by changing the subject or asking a question back!
7. If the interview is being broadcast 'live' be careful what you say. If it is being recorded, don't be afraid to ask to repeat part of the interview.

Combining mass media with face-to-face education

Mass media will have more impact if it is combined with face-to-face communication. When people listen to radio programmes or read newspapers they usually discuss the content with others in their family or community. This natural process can be built upon in your health education programme. For example, you can brief your fieldworkers in advance so that they follow up broadcasts with discussions with the community in clinics, on home visits or at meetings.

People often listen to radio in groups. You can deliberately encourage this by setting up a *radio listening group* – or 'radio forum'. This would consist of between 10 and 20 people who may either be an existing group in the community or one specially set up, such as a group of mothers at a health centre. A group leader introduces the programme and, after listening to the programme, a discussion is held on the content. Experience with radio listening groups suggest the following guidelines.

- Use visual aids such as posters or a flip chart to help the discussion. They can be shown to the group during the radio programme to emphasise key points, add a visual dimension and assist the discussion at the end. Provide leaflets for the audience to take away.
- Ask the group questions to make them think about the programme and the key messages. Note their comments and send them back to the programme organisers. This provides valuable feedback on the relevance of the programme and the needs of the communities.
- Mobilise other workers in the community to help you. School teachers and fieldworkers from health, agriculture, family-planning and literacy services could lead the listening groups. You can provide simple training to introduce the health topics, use the visual aids and simple group discussion skills.

An early example of the use of the radio forum is the *Mtu ni afya* campaign that took place in 1973 in Tanzania. In this campaign

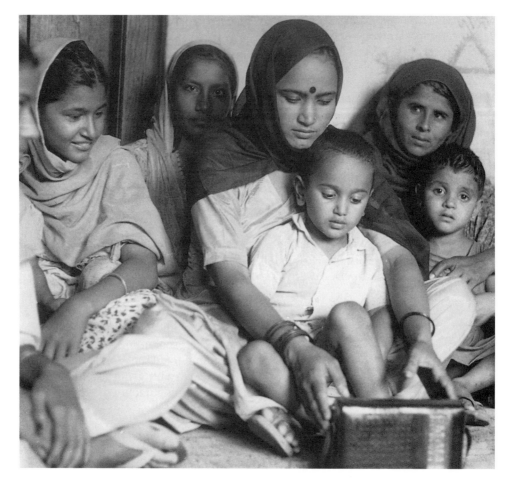

Fig. 8.3   Radio learning group in Haryana State, India

twelve 30-minute radio programmes were each broadcast twice a week over a 12-week period. Through an intensive programme of seminars, 75,000 study-group leaders were trained and an estimated 2 million participants listened to the broadcasts in study groups. A manual was produced for the group leaders, study guides for the participants and a series of flip charts to be used during the broadcasts. The first 10 minutes of each radio programme consisted of an introductory signature tune, news about the progress of the campaign and songs and poems. A study of health practices before and after the campaign showed some limited changes in health practices including use of latrines.

Botswana is another African country that has used radio forums. Figure 8.4 is taken from their excellent handbook on designing radio forums. Even if you cannot produce your own radio programmes you can still use this approach in your community. Any health broadcast provides an opportunity for a group to meet. If there is a regular broadcast on health you can arrange for a group to meet and listen to it. You can write and find out in advance the topics to be covered and prepare suitable discussion questions.

Audio cassettes

One disadvantage with radio is that the time of broadcast may not be very convenient for the group. This problem is easily overcome by recording the programme on a cassette recorder

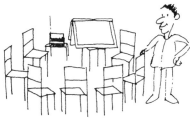

1. prepare the meeting place and study materials

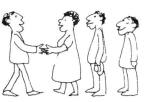

2. welcome the members

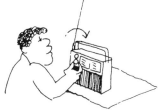

3. turn on the radio

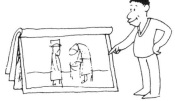

4. refer to the flipchart pictures

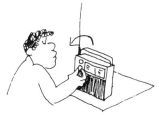

5. turn off the radio

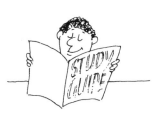

6. read the study guide

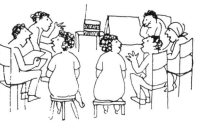

7. discuss each question

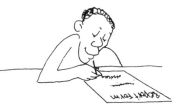

8. fill in the report form

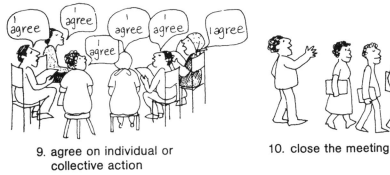

9. agree on individual or collective action

10. close the meeting

Fig. 8.4   Organising radio listening groups in Botswana

so the group can listen to it at a time that suits everyone. This has many advantages:

- You are not restricted to a particular broadcast time.
- Broadcast programmes can be used repeatedly with many groups (but be careful of copyright laws).

- You can stop the cassette during the programme, repeat sections and discuss points when they arise.

Radio suffers from the disadvantage that programmes are directed at the general population and do not meet the specific needs of local groups. However it is not difficult to record locally relevant health education programmes on cassettes. These can be played to local audiences while waiting at clinics, to groups of women in workshops, through public address systems in villages, markets, on top of vehicles and other locations.

An example of this was a health education project in Guatemala carried out by Colle and co-workers. They carried out a small research study on the lifestyle and needs of the women in the community. This study identified their concerns and present practices, and showed that most women spent some time in the week at a public laundry facility. They recorded a health education programme which used an entertaining magazine format that included drama, music and talks. Members of the community were paid to play the cassettes at the public laundry facilities and change the cassettes regularly. A different programme was prepared for each day during a 3-week period. An evaluation of the impact of the programme showed improvements both in knowledge and adoption of health practices.

Practical broadcasting techniques

You do not need sophisticated equipment to produce simple programmes for your own community. But it is worth making your recordings to a high as standard as possible. If they are good enough, radio stations will be prepared to broadcast them to reach a wide audience. The experienced radio broadcaster Maggie Mash has suggested the guidelines below as well as the 'Tips for being interviewed' on page 149 and 'Guidelines for good broadcasting' on page 154.

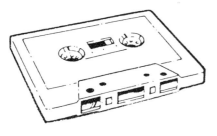

Fig. 8.5 An audio cassette

Case studies of the use of mass media

Using mass media to motivate men to go for vasectomies in Sao Paolo, Brazil. Four advertisements ran for 10 weeks in eight magazines – 18 advertisements in weekly magazines and nine in monthly magazines with an estimated target readership of 4.4 million men over 30 years of age. Clients coming to clinics doubled during the campaign and 18% of the new clients arriving during the campaign period reported having seen one of the magazine advertisements.

A 7-month national mass media campaign to promote immunisation in the Philippines. The mass media campaign consisted of four television and four radio advertisements and advertisements placed in newspapers. Other promotional materials included: posters, welcome streamers, stickers, T-shirts. The campaign slogan 'Protect your baby from measles' and messages emphasised that vaccinations were free and available on Wednesday at health centres. City mayors, health officers and clinic staff were briefed before the campaign. The percentage of fully immunised children increased from 54% to 65%.

Mental health promotion using television in South Africa. The South African Broadcasting Corporation screened a TV series called 'Improve Your Frames of Mind', which focused on the signs and symptoms of the main psychiatric disorders. At the end of each show, the telephone number of a mental health information centre was given. Almost 3000 calls with requests for information on psychiatric disorders were received.

Immunisation campaign in Mexico. The National Vaccination Council launched three immunisation campaigns for polio and measles every year. Messages targeted at both adults and children are broadcast on radio and television. Most of the messages are based on popular children's songs or slogans. TV spots used cartoons or animated clay figures. In addition posters, flyers, newspaper ads and announcements were widely used. Private companies, NGOs and schools participated in the campaign – notifying parents of the campaign. Face-to-face motivation of mothers was also given by health workers or volunteers at the immunisation posts or during home visits. An evaluation found that more than half of a sample of mothers interviewed were aware of the campaign and its purpose. Mothers who were aware of the campaign were more likely to have brought their children for immunisation than those who had not seen the campaign.

Leprosy education programme in Madras, India. Posters with the message 'Leprosy is curable' were placed on the entire fleet of city buses in Madras city. A total of 500 interviews were done at major bus stands, terminals and busy traffic junctions. All the respondents had seen the posters and could correctly describe the message it displayed. Three-quarters made positive comments about the curability of leprosy and the need to remove stigma and just over half said that they would like to know more about leprosy.

Male motivation radio campaign in Zimbabwe. The campaign consisted of a 52-episode radio soap opera broadcast twice a week, 60 educational talks to groups of between 12 and several hundred men in mines, farms, factories and villages, and two pamphlets about contraceptive methods. A follow-up survey showed that the campaign reached just over half of all men aged 18 to 55. Among married Shona-speaking men, use of modern contraceptive methods increased from about 56% to 59% and condom use increased from about 5% to 10%.

Mass media promotion of breastfeeding in Jordan. Two intensive radio and television campaigns each lasting about 2 months were carried out using drama, testimonials and advice from a fictitious female doctor. Messages included : 'initiate breastfeeding within the first hours after birth', the benefits of colostrum, that breast milk is all the child needs for the first 4 months of life, and advice on some common breastfeeding problems. The evaluation found that the mass media had a positive impact on mothers' knowledge of the importance of colostrum and breastfeeding, and also increased the initiation of breastfeeding at home and in public hospitals.

Posters and video to promote malaria uptake of treatment in Cambodia. One hundred and fifty posters were distributed in each of two groups of villages for display in schools, temples, clinics, pharmacies, village chief's offices, army camps, plantation units and video parlours. In one group of villages videos were shown approximately 25–30 times each week in video parlours, restaurants and at ceremonial gatherings. Drug sellers and health care workers in both groups of villages were trained on the importance of giving advice to encourage adherence to prescribed medicines. In the villages where only posters were used, adherence to malaria medication rose from 6% to 11%. An even greater effect was found in the villages receiving both video and posters when the rates of adherence increased to 20%.

A mass media health education campaign for TB control in Cali, Colombia. The 6-week media campaign had three components; the television and radio components consisted of public service announcements and chat shows involving people with tuberculosis, doctors and heath educators; the printed component consisted of leaflets inserted in local newspapers and feature articles in newspapers. The purpose of the campaign was to reduce levels of prejudice against people with TB and motivate people to come for diagnosis and treatment. Following the campaign the number of direct smears processed by the laboratories increased by 64% and the number of confirmed new cases of TB increased by 52%. However, the improvements did not continue after the radio campaign ended – pointing to the need for continuing media support.

The tape recorder

This is the essential tool of the trade. Portable tape recorders are usually battery operated. Always test the tape recorder before you take it anywhere – and test it again before starting to record! After finishing a recording it is always a good idea to play back a few seconds to make sure it has recorded. Take adequate supplies of tapes and batteries. High quality programmes are usually made on 'reel-to-reel' recorders but good quality recordings can also be made on cassette recorders that are simpler to operate. The best recorders have controls for sound levels that you can adjust according to the volume of the sound you are recording. However most ordinary cassette machines have automatic level controls which are easier to use – but cannot produce special effects such as 'fading' music at the end of a programme.

The microphone

The secret to a good recording is to use a microphone. Avoid using the built-in microphones on cassette recorders as they tend to pick up the sound of the machinery of the cassette recorder. Keep the microphone about 6 inches from the mouth of the person speaking. It is best to have the microphone on a stand. If you do hold it by hand, wrap the cable around your fingers so the cable doesn't make a noise when you move. If you are recording outside, wind can be a problem: try to record in a protected area, such as underneath a coat with your back to the wind. If it is very noisy turn the recording level down and hold the microphone closer. If a room echoes, turn the recording level down and hold the microphone closer. Try not to move the microphone too much. If recording music, position the microphone nearer the voice(s) than the instrument and hold the microphone further away than for speech. The above are only rough guides. It is always best to try recording a

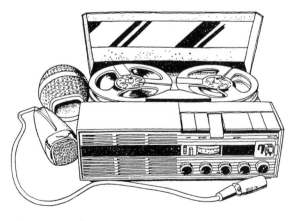

Fig. 8.6   Reel-to-reel recorder

little bit and play back the recording to find out if it sounds right.

Editing

This is the process by which you can remove unwanted parts of a recording such as background noises, unnecessary questions and mistakes and join several different recordings together to make a programme. Tape from a reel-to-reel recording can be edited by cutting the tape and joining together the parts that you want. 'Dub' editing is a simpler process by which you connect two recorders and record the different parts you want from the original recordings onto a 'master' tape.

Guidelines on good broadcasting

1. **Be brief**: Assume the listener gets bored easily and can very easily 'switch off' mentally or physically at any time.
2. **Be entertaining**: Above all the listener wants to be entertained by the broadcast; make it as lively and interesting as possible. Try to make the message more acceptable by use of music, comedy or drama. Don't lecture.
3. **Be clear**: It is no use burying the message too far in the entertainment, or making it obscure. Be simple, use straightforward ordinary language (local dialect). In a book it is always possible to read a section again if you do not understand it first time. You can't do this with radio or television so it is a good idea to repeat the message at different times in the programme. Speak clearly and don't rush. Addresses, dates and phone numbers (and any important names or numbers) should always be repeated.
4. **Aim for maximum impact**: Always try to start a programme with something that catches the attention, e.g. baby crying, music, jingle, crash, or a striking word or question. End with something that people will remember.
5. **Dialogue or discussion** is always more interesting than only one person talking. It is very difficult to hold attention with one voice.
6. **Aim for variety**: Don't put in too much speech or very long pieces of music. Try putting

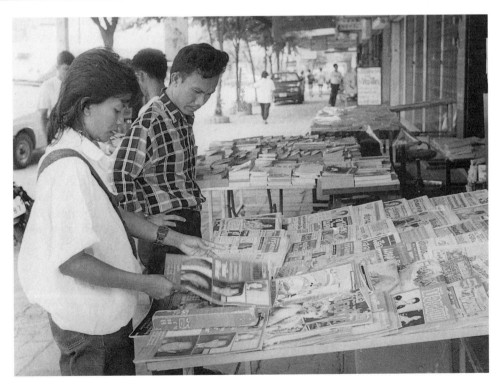

a music background to the speech, use different voices, ask questions; keep the listeners guessing what will come next; try not to be predictable.

7. ***Choose carefully the people you interview***. When interviewing or choosing participants for discussion programmes *choose your people carefully*. They also must speak clearly and simply and be interesting.

8. ***Put 'colour' into interviews***: Create a picture in the mind of your listeners that will help them to set the interview into its situation. Describe your surroundings, the family, the area, and what's going on.

9. ***Ask 'how' and 'why' questions*** that allow people to express ideas and opinions; avoid questions that just need the yes or no answers.

10. ***Write for the listener or viewer***: Always think of one person the other side of the microphone and address them personally, as you would a friend. Be confidential with them and conversational. Say 'you' and 'we', not 'listeners'. Use the colloquial language of ordinary people.

Print media

Newspapers and magazines can be a useful way of reaching the community with your health education messages. Obviously you will only be able to reach those who can read and can afford to buy them. But that audience will often include opinion leaders and influential persons.

Leaflets

These are the most common way of using print media in health education. The simplest leaflet is a single sheet of paper, printed on both sides, and folded in half or into thirds. Leaflets can be larger with two or more sheets of paper. Once there are more than five sheets it is common to use the term 'booklet'. Leaflets can be a useful reinforcement for individual and group sessions and serve as a reminder of the main points that you have made. Even if people cannot read, they can ask others to read them for them. Leaflets are helpful for sensitive subjects such as

Fig. 8.7   Magazines on sale in Thailand

sex when people are too shy to ask but can pick up a leaflet and read the information.

Suitable leaflets may already be available for your health education work. However, leaflets produced by others may not be directly relevant, either because of language or content so you may have to produce leaflets for your own community. However, these do not have to be expensively produced to a sophisticated standard – especially if the topic is one that your target readership is interested in.

A useful starting point is to look at leaflets produced in other programmes in your country or from abroad. This will give you ideas on how you can adapt the ideas to your own situation. Make the language simple with pictures and try out draft versions to make sure that they are understood. Always include an address where people can go for further information. Give them out at talks or counselling sessions, leave them in public places and make them available on demand after a radio or television programme. Think of places in the community where you can leave the leaflets and people might come across them. Look out for opportunities to distribute them in different ways such as wage packets, voters' registrations forms, electricity bills and rent statements etc. A simple check list that you can use for testing out a leaflet is:

- Is it interesting to look at?
- Does it contain relevant information for the target readership?
- Does it avoid distracting irrelevant information?
- Is the language easy to read?
- Does it avoid complicated technical words?
- Is the advice presented realistic and feasible?
- Does it provide the specific information that the target audience actually want to know?
- Does it tell people where they can get further information?

Magazines

Some health educators have tried producing their own health magazine. For example in India a voluntary organisation, the Catholic Hospital Association of India, produces a magazine called *Health Action*. This covers a range of health topics in a visually attractive way and is sold through newspaper outlets. In Zimbabwe, a children's comic called *Action* covers a range of health and environmental issues (see Figure 9.8 in the next chapter). Producing your own magazine is an exciting idea but needs careful thought and preparation. If you plan to give it away through health clinics and schools you will need to obtain funding on a regular basis. You might be able to cover part of the costs of production through selling advertising to local companies. The challenge would be to sell it commercially through shops and newspaper stands so that it pays for itself. If people have paid for it they are more likely to read and value it than if you simply gave it to them free. However, if you do plan to sell the magazine, it must be well produced and entertaining so that people are prepared to pay money for it.

In parts of Latin America *photo novellas* are popular. These are story books of photographs with accompanying dialogue. In Asia, similar books are widely popular using drawings and text. In Burma a story book was prepared where the theme of leprosy was built into a dramatic story. It was written and drawn by local writers and artists and the finished book was sold alongside other story books and widely distributed. In Thailand a story book on hygiene has been produced.

Producing your own magazine is a big task. You may not have the time or resources to take this on – then it would be better to try to interest existing magazines in covering health topics. Most of what was discussed above about influencing the media, writing press releases and staging media events is also relevant to magazines. Try to find out who reads the different newspapers and magazines. There may be specialist magazines aimed at reaching young people, businessmen and women that could be suited for your needs.

Some tips on clear writing

Whether you are writing the words for a poster, leaflet, newspaper article, or story book you will have to pay attention to your writing style. In looking at written materials we usually separate out two concepts:

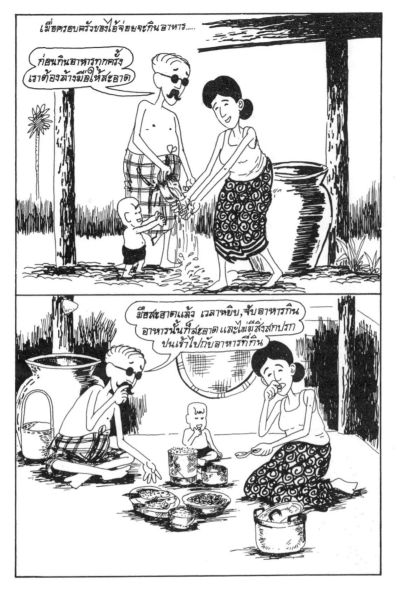

Fig. 8.8   Picture story book on hygiene from Thailand

- *Legibility* refers to whether the actual words can be distinguished on the paper; writing which is too faint, too small, uses complicated typefaces or where the ink has smudged are all difficult to read.
- *Readability* refers to how easy it is to understand the meaning of the text: too many unfamiliar words, long sentences, complicated sentence structures with different sections, long paragraphs, crowded pages, and no headings can all make text difficult to understand.

Just because a piece of writing is clear to you does not mean that others will also understand it. Young children may still be developing their reading skills. Your audience may have left school early or have only learnt to read as adults. The written material may even be in the community's second language or be written in a different style. For example, in India a translation was made of the WHO publication *The Primary Health Care Worker* from English into Hindi. An evaluation study showed that the book was not understood because the language used was a formal style using 'polite' expressions rather than everyday ordinary language. Many health education writings were originally written in English and you should be careful to translate them with appropriate language. This can be difficult as the language may not have local equivalents for technical words. If you have translated something from English it is always a good idea to ask someone else to translate the text back into English and see if it has kept the meaning.

Writing in simple language is not easy. It is worth studying the style used by newspapers, magazines and books that are read by your community. See if you can adopt their language, choice of words and general approach. Each language will have its own rules about writing clearly and simply and some tips on clear writing are given here.

Some tips on clear writing in English

- Write simply; avoid using a 'literary' style.
- Keep sentences short; avoid long sentences with too many sections; vary the length of sentences to keep the writing interesting.
- Use simple words that are understood by the intended audience; avoid abbreviations and technical words; if you use specialised words, make sure you explain them.
- Use active rather than passive forms of verbs – use 'poor hygiene causes diarrhoea' rather than 'diarrhoea is caused by poor hygiene'.
- Lay the text out on the page to make it easy to read – avoid crowding the page with writing – space it out.
- Use lists and 'bullets' (a dots or symbol in front of each point as in with this list) to bring out main points.
- Avoid small print and fancy typefaces; use headlines, **bold** letters, *italics* to emphasise different sections and important words; keep the use of capital ('upper case') letters to a minimum.
- Use diagrams and pictures to explain ideas; put them close to the part of the text they refer to; make sure that they can be easily understood by the reader.

Posters

Posters can range in size from large billboards to small notices. Production of posters has dominated the work of many health education services. They have been given too much emphasis, compared with more effective approaches such as community mobilisation, drama, group teaching and one-to-one counselling. By themselves posters have little value. They are useful mainly to bring a topic to the attention of the community, reinforce a message that the public is receiving through other channels such as radio and face-to-face and provide a talking point for discussion. Examples of appropriate use include posters:

- used to reinforce the main theme of a radio campaign;
- used in a clinic as the theme for a talk;
- put up in a village to draw attention to a community meeting; and
- outside a shop to say that condoms are available.

Some of the issues involved in the design and use of use of posters, including the content, visual perception, and choice of location were discussed in Chapter 3. A good poster should have a very simple message and not try to say too much. Unlike a wallchart, which is a learning aid to accompany a lesson, a poster has to be clear enough to be understood on its own. It should be 'eye catching' – gaining attention by use of striking pictures, bright colours or interesting content.

Posters should be displayed where your intended audience will pass them and see them. There is no point in just displaying them at clinics where they will only be seen by a small group of people. You will need to use different locations, depending on the intended audience, e.g. young people, men, pregnant women, long-distance drivers, soldiers. Do not leave the same one up for too long as people will become familiar with it and not notice it.

Other print media

Calendars are another popular print medium. They can show the days of the month and health education messages. If it is attractive, people will hang it up in their home and workplace. The new page every month provides a way of regularly changing the message and matching it to the season.

Postage stamps have been used by many countries including Tanzania, Bangladesh and Sri Lanka to carry health education messages.

Combining entertainment and mass media

The potential of popular media was shown in the previous chapter. In recent years there has been increasing interest in using entertainment programmes in the mass media to promote health. One of the best known examples has been the *Soul City* television drama series from South Africa and 'soap operas' using a similar storytelling format have been launched in many other countries, especially on radio. The challenge with this approach is to obtain the right balance between entertainment and education. It is important to allow enough time for the characters to become established before introducing health issues. A typical approach is to contrast the behaviours of different characters in

a story, e.g. a character who does all the wrong things and as a result has poor health. Another approach is to have misfortune strike a character, who then takes appropriate action to deal with their problem. Launching a new soap opera is a major task involving considerable outlay in time, money and expertise. A simpler approach is to try to interest the producers of existing television and radio entertainment programmes to introduce health issues into their storylines.

The Internet and health promotion

The Internet is a network of computers throughout the world. All that is required to use the Internet is a computer, a telephone line and a local service provider. Once you are connected you can 'log on' and 'browse' a vast number of 'web sites' and the information they contain. Access to the Internet is still quite limited in many countries but widespread in the industrialised world where more and more people working in health promotion have started to use this new medium for:

• provision of specialist information on health topics;

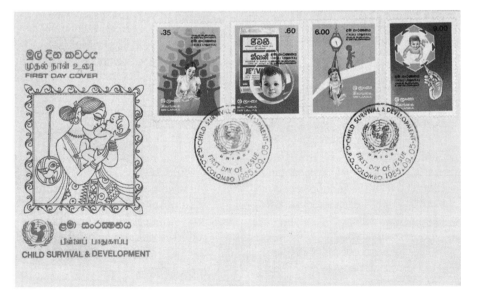

Fig. 8.9   Postage stamps on health from Sri Lanka

Examples of combining entertainment and mass media

Radio soap opera in Tanzania. A radio soap opera *Twende na Wakati* (Let's go with the times) was broadcast in Kiswahili twice a week for 30 minutes over a 6-year period from July 1993. Four key HIV/AIDS prevention themes were covered: (1) that STDs should be treated; (2) that condoms can prevent HIV infection; (3) that AIDS is an incurable disease that is spread by sexual contact; and (4) that the rumours about AIDS are false. The characters in the soap operas were designed to provide both negative and positive role models for HIV prevention behaviours, as well as examples of people undergoing change in their approach to risk. An evaluation found that the programme was listened to by more than half of the target population and that there was a decrease in reported number of sexual contacts in districts receiving the broadcasts compared with those that did not receive them.

Promotion of family planning in Ilorin, Ibadan and Enugu cities in Nigeria. Family planning dramas were included in existing popular television entertainment shows in a 3-year campaign. Also four radio spots were broadcast 169 times; five television spots were broadcast 110 times; two newspaper advertisements were published for 6 weeks; and 1500 copies six posters were displayed. An estimated half of the population had watched the programmes. Following the media promotion the number of new clinic clients per quarter increased in all cities by amounts which varied from two times (Ilorin) to increases of five times (Enugu).

'Sparrows don't migrate' family planning mass media campaign in Turkey. Focus-group discussions among women were used to generate campaign message themes for a 3-month intensive campaign using television spots and documentaries supported by radio and print media. Extensive use was made of humour, music and emotional drama. An evaluation survey showed that: 80% of married women were exposed to the campaign; 63% said that they had talked to their husbands about family planning; 10% of married women said they had visited a family planning clinic as a result of the

campaign; and a further 20% said that they intended to make a visit. Family planning clinics reported an increase in contraceptive uptake.

Mass media and family planning in The Gambia. The campaign consisted of 30-second radio spots and a 39-episode radio drama. Messages were designed to convey the beliefs that Islam supports the use of modern contraception, that the modern methods are safe, that family planning service providers are knowledgeable and caring, and that couples should discuss family planning. An evaluation found that people who had heard the serial drama could name significantly more contraceptive methods; were significantly more positive about family planning; and were also more likely to use a modern method than those who had not heard the drama.

Multimedia campaign to promote family planning in Tanzania. The 2-year multimedia campaign relied on radio spots, a radio serial drama called *Zinduca*, a logo, posters, leaflets, newspapers, audio cassettes and television. An evaluation found that 55% of women had been exposed to family planning messages in the previous 6 months. Radio was the medium that had had the widest impact – 49% had heard family planning messages from radio, 23% of women had seen family planning messages in newspapers, 18% from posters, 8% from leaflets and only 4% from television. Use of modern contraceptive methods was far greater among women who recalled family planning messages that among those who did not.

- self-help guides on health topics;
- a point of contact for questions on health;
- a way of getting in touch with people having similar health concerns;
- on-line 'health appraisals' where a person can answer questions about lifestyle including sexual behaviour, diet, exercise and alcohol consumption and then receive a personalised report about their health status and actions they can take to reduce risks.

The Internet has been used to reach young people who are especially receptive to new approaches and may prefer to obtain information from a computer than to approach an adult. Surprisingly, people can find it more comfortable talking to an anonymous computer about their personal lives than speaking to a real person who they feel might pass judgement.

As our experience of this exciting new medium grows, some lessons are beginning to appear. Its effectiveness depends on a person making the effort to use their own computer to log onto a web site – so the information provided on a web site only reaches people who are actively searching for information or help on a topic. One of the strengths of the Internet is that it is interactive. A person is able to select information that matches his or her needs. If a web site is not clearly laid out and does not contain information a person wants, he or she will not bother to look at the web site or will quickly move to other places on the Internet. A typical search on the Internet can easily yield thousands of sites providing information on a health topic. It is easy to become overwhelmed by this vast amount of information. Another concern is that the information provided on the Internet is not monitored for accuracy or quality so that it is possible that people may receive incorrect, biased or misleading information. This is especially true with web sites that are set up by commercial companies who are trying to sell their product.

The Internet is emerging as a major resource for those involved in designing and implementing health promotion activities – providing access to research findings and opportunities for sharing information with other practitioners. At the end of this book you will find a list of some web sites that provide useful resources for health promotion. Its contribution as a medium for directly reaching out to members of the community is still far from clear.

Some conclusions on using mass media

If well-planned, mass media can be an extremely powerful way of promoting health in your community. They can have an impact on their own as well as create a favourable climate of understanding and concern for a topic that field-workers can take advantage of in their face-to-face work. Even if you do not have access to facilities and resources for preparing your own programmes, you can still encourage the media to take up health issues. Some characteristics of different media are shown in Figure 8.11.

The 'P' approach in Figure 8.10 is a helpful guide to remembering the steps in preparing media communication. It was developed by the Population Communication Centre at Johns Hopkins University in the United States, which has played a leading role in social marketing and entertainment-based mass media health promotion programmes in developing countries.

Summary

The following guidelines summarise the main points in this chapter.

1 Decide at the outset what can be realistically achieved by each medium and what cannot. Aim for what can be achieved. Set specific, measurable objectives.
2 Learn lessons from similar campaigns elsewhere and make sure that you do not repeat their mistakes.
3 Base your programme on an analysis of the health issue and its causes. Make sure that the advice you give is accurate, relevant and feasible.
4 Decide which sections of the public you are trying to reach and find out what media they watch, listen to and read. Carry out a simple study on what they believe, feel and know about the health issue. Use this information to make the message specific to the particular audience's needs and to decide on the timing, location and content of your activities.
5 Make friends with journalists and media producers. If you can provide them with interesting stories they will report your activities and provide free publicity.
6 Make your programmes entertaining and avoid 'preaching'. Include popular media such as songs, drama, puppets (see Chapter 7). If you are using dramas and stories,

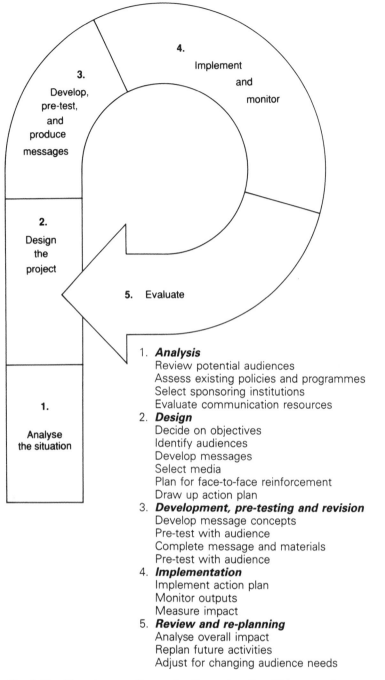

1. **Analysis**
   Review potential audiences
   Assess existing policies and programmes
   Select sponsoring institutions
   Evaluate communication resources
2. **Design**
   Decide on objectives
   Identify audiences
   Develop messages
   Select media
   Plan for face-to-face reinforcement
   Draw up action plan
3. **Development, pre-testing and revision**
   Develop message concepts
   Pre-test with audience
   Complete message and materials
   Pre-test with audience
4. **Implementation**
   Implement action plan
   Monitor outputs
   Measure impact
5. **Review and re-planning**
   Analyse overall impact
   Replan future activities
   Adjust for changing audience needs

Fig. 8.10   Planning media production using the 'P' approach
(Population Communication Services, Johns Hopkins University)

build up the characters and human interest first before including health messages. Wherever possible, involve people with experience in media in producing pro-

grammes. Use sources that are trusted by the community.

7 Do not put too many messages into each programme. Always pre-test your pro-

grammes and messages with a sample of the target audience before they are broadcast to make sure they are properly understood and accepted.

8 Broadcast programmes as often as possible. Make them available in other formats – distribute the radio programme on audio cassettes, the TV programme on video, the newspaper article as a leaflet.

9 Try to identify person-to-person advice systems in the community that you could mobilise to reinforce your media activities. Hold discussions with them before the campaign and, if necessary, arrange for some training. Provide written materials to accompany the broadcasts such as a leaflet.

10 When you use radio or television, prepare reinforcing media such as listening guides, workbooks, simple booklets. A multimedia approach usually will do better than a single channel.

11 Always include a way by which the audience can obtain help or further information, e.g. an address to write to or telephone.

12 Try to build in some mechanism for audience feedback, e.g. letters, and include some method of evaluation. In the short term you should try to find out how many watched, heard or read the programmes and understood the messages. In the longer term you can find out if people remembered the message, accepted the advice and if any change in behaviour took place.

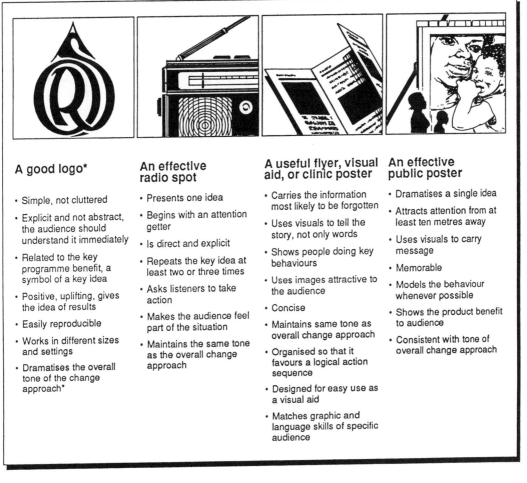

A good logo*

- Simple, not cluttered
- Explicit and not abstract, the audience should understand it immediately
- Related to the key programme benefit, a symbol of a key idea
- Positive, uplifting, gives the idea of results
- Easily reproducible
- Works in different sizes and settings
- Dramatises the overall tone of the change approach*

An effective radio spot

- Presents one idea
- Begins with an attention getter
- Is direct and explicit
- Repeats the key idea at least two or three times
- Asks listeners to take action
- Makes the audience feel part of the situation
- Maintains the same tone as the overall change approach

A useful flyer, visual aid, or clinic poster

- Carries the information most likely to be forgotten
- Uses visuals to tell the story, not only words
- Shows people doing key behaviours
- Uses images attractive to the audience
- Concise
- Maintains same tone as overall change approach
- Organised so that it favours a logical action sequence
- Designed for easy use as a visual aid
- Matches graphic and language skills of specific audience

An effective public poster

- Dramatises a single idea
- Attracts attention from at least ten metres away
- Uses visuals to carry message
- Memorable
- Models the behaviour whenever possible
- Shows the product benefit to audience
- Consistent with tone of overall change approach

Fig. 8.11   Characteristics of media

9 Working with children and young people

Almost half the population of most developing countries is made up of children under 15. In carrying out education and communication programmes with children and young people we usually have two broad objectives in mind: the first is to improve the health of the children and young people themselves; the second is to provide the knowledge, attitudes and skills to prepare them for their future lives. This chapter will examine:

1 the special considerations that need to be taken when directing health education at children and young people;
2 how schools can be used to promote health of young children and future adults;
3 how communication programmes can reach young people out of school.

Special considerations with children and young people

In Chapter 4 you were introduced to the approaches involved in carrying out education and training activities with adults. However, an adult will have fully developed thinking powers and a wide range of experiences to contribute to the learning. Different approaches are needed in educational programmes for children. Children are still *developing*. Depending on his or her age, a child will still be developing his or her understanding of themselves, other people and the world around them.

The period of life between birth and 20 years is one of enormous change. These changes include *physical, intellectual, social and emotional development*. Think about your own experiences with the following groups: children between birth and 5 years (under fives or pre-school children), the primary school aged child (5 to 11), and the older child from 11 to 16 years. How would you adapt your approach, teaching methods, content and language to each of these groups?

Physical development

Growth in weight and size are the most obvious physical changes. In addition, as children grow they can perform increasingly more complex tasks with their hands and show greater coordination and strength in their movements. From about 10–13 years onwards the sexual organs develop, as do secondary sexual characteristics of pubic and facial hair and changes in the voice.

Disease, malnutrition and injuries from accidents and violence can affect physical development and lead to reduced growth ('stunting'), deformities and various forms of disability. Good physical development is promoted by a safe environment, adequate diet, preventive health care measures, and opportunities for practising skills involving movement, coordination and handling of objects.

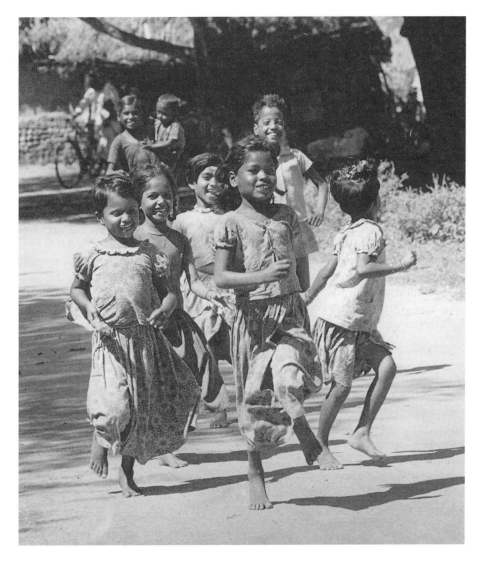

Fig. 9.1   Children

Social, emotional and language development

At birth a baby is dependent on the people around him or her, especially the mother. As a child becomes older he/she interacts with others in the family and through this develops language, beliefs, values, concepts and behaviours that make up the culture of the family, community and society. Important components of social development are the abilities to form relation-ships, communicate and cooperate with other people. Also important, is the development of our ideas about who we are, what we can do, what our future might be. 'Self-concept' is the word used to describe the sum total of our ideas about who we think we are. Our judgement and feelings about whether we feel that we are worthwhile is called 'self-esteem'.

This early learning from within the family is called *primary socialisation*. Later, a child begins to be exposed to influences outside the family including friends, teachers, books, radio and television, and this is called *secondary socialisation*. In later childhood and during adolescence, friends – called the 'peer' group are extremely influential. Anything that affects the stability of the family and relationships with friends can have a damaging effect on social and emotional development. This can include break-up of families from disease, war, family violence, alcohol and influences of poverty and unemployment.

Social and emotional development are promoted by a combination of measures. These include: social and economic measures that give families the resources to maintain their stability and provide the caring environment for their children; advice and help to families on caring for their children; and services providing good quality care for children separated from their parents for short or longer periods, such as in pre-school facilities or orphanages.

Intellectual development

Intellectual or 'cognitive' development is concerned with how the growing child develops the ability to *think*. This includes processes of perceiving and building up a mental picture of the surrounding world. It also includes the ability to draw on concepts, rules and procedures to solve problems and make decisions. At the beginning of primary school a child may think in more 'concrete' or specific ways tied to the appearance of things and may only have a limited ability for abstract thinking. As children get older, they develop a greater ability to think in abstract ways, apply concepts, symbols and rules to solve problems. An older child will also have more experiences within and outside the family that can be used to help his or her understanding of the world.

Many factors affect intellectual development. A child has a natural curiosity about the world. The more this curiosity is stimulated with discussions, questions and activities as well as experiences such as visits to interesting places, the more the child's intellect will be developed. Malnutrition and illness have a harmful effect on the way children learn. A hungry child will

be tired, inactive and find it difficult to concentrate. Serious malnutrition can lead to permanent disabilities such as blindness and stunting of growth. Illnesses also prevent children from attending school and affect their ability to concentrate and learn. Disabilities such as poor hearing, eyesight and physical movement also affect a child's ability to learn.

Because of the various influences on intellectual development described above, it is not surprising that poverty, poor living conditions and large family size can have a harmful effect on intellectual development. But encouragement of intellectual development of children is not just a matter of meeting needs for food, housing and health care. These physical needs should be supplemented by providing a stimulating and challenging environment. Learning opportunities in the family, community, pre-school and school environment can all help a child to achieve his or her potential.

Adolescence

In recent years concern about drugs, alcohol, solvent abuse, smoking and teenage pregnancies have led to greater attention on the period of adolescence. Adolescence involves the following changes:

- *biological changes* body size and proportions;
- *development of sexuality* both physical and emotional; sexual organs and secondary sexual characteristics such as hair, breasts;
- *development of ideas about one's identity and future roles* with possible conflict with expectations of one's family and community.

A biological approach would define adolescence as the time when the human being acquires the ability to reproduce. Another approach is to view adolescence as the period of transition between being a child and acquiring adult status. In traditional societies the period of childhood can be quite short and even quite young children have responsibilities, working in the home and in agricultural work. Special ceremonies of initiation often marked the point when the child becomes the adult. These ceremonies showed public recognition that the children were adults and often included practical instruction on adult behaviour and sex education.

In Western industrialised societies the period of transition to adult roles is later. During the period up to 16 years a young person is still considered a child, is not allowed to carry out adult work and still attends school. Teenage pregnancy can lead to leaving school early and prevent opportunities for further education. For most children the period of adolescence passes without any problems. For some, it can be a difficult stage – of 'storm and stress' – with conflict, rebellion and disagreements with parents and teachers. This conflict can show itself in experimentation with sex, drugs, smoking and alcohol.

Most developing countries are experiencing rapid social change, urbanisation, and increased exposure to mass media. Traditional systems are rapidly changing, initiation ceremonies are less common and increasingly children are staying on at school. Adolescence in many developing countries is beginning to resemble the situation in industrialised countries.

The pre-school child

As I described above, the first 5 years of a child's life are extremely important for the development of the child. The foundations of physical, intellectual, social, emotional and language development are being laid. Health education can be carried out with the pre-school child in many ways. One important way is through educational programmes reaching the 'caretakers' of the child. These caretakers might include the parents – usually the mother – and other members of the family involved in decision-making on child care including the father, grandparents or older brother and sister. Educational programmes can involve:

- family life education provided in schools for preparing pupils for future roles as parents;
- education on child care and child development provided for parents as part of antenatal education or at child health clinics;

- non-formal education of parents in the home and community settings such as women's groups, fathers' clubs, churches and other organisations; and
- public education directed at families involving various forms of media including books, leaflets, magazine articles, radio and television programmes providing advice on parenthood.

It is possible to reach pre-school children directly through crèches or nurseries. These might be run by government, private and voluntary agencies and provide care and support for children for all or part of the day. Some nurseries are able to care for very young children from the first few months. Others do not take children until they are 2–3 years old. Crèches and nurseries can benefit the health and development of the pre-school child in many ways as shown in Figure 9.2

Many people think that learning must always involve formal 'teaching' sessions. They treat play as a way of keeping a child amused, filling in time and do not consider it very important. However, one of the most important ways in which pre-school children develop is through play. While playing, children learn new things including: exploring movements by using hands and the body and balancing; developing powers of thinking; finding out how to express themselves; using imagination; and learning how to get on with others.

Play is an activity that takes place naturally. For example, even in traditional rural communities, it is common to see young children playing at adult roles with pretend stoves and dolls. Most children have curiosity and interest in the world around them. Without any special effort they will involve the people around them and make use of whatever objects they come into contact with such as leaves, twigs and household objects.

If play is such a natural process, why then do we need to need to make a special effort to promote it? Parents and services are often unaware of how their children's development can be helped through play. The most important resource is the willingness of adults to spend time doing things with young

Pre-school provisions improve child health and development by

{

enabling mothers to work and increase family income

releasing young girls from child care duties so that they can attend school

providing opportunities for reaching children with child health and nutrition services including screening, growth monitoring, immunisation, child-feeding programmes

educational opportunities (e.g. for social, emotional, language and intellectual development) for children from poor and deprived communities and laying the foundations for good performance at school

specific health education activities which encourage healthy routines such as handwashing, care of teeth, nutrition

providing opportunities to carry out non-formal education with parents on child health and development

Fig. 9.2   Ways in which pre-school provisions can improve child health and development

children – it is not necessary to spend large amounts of money on expensive toys to promote play. It is possible to make simple and very effective 'junk toys' from every-day items such as plastic bottles and cardboard boxes. Verbal play can involve storytelling, riddles and jokes. Pre-school provisions such as crèches can provide an even wider range of experiences than the home and can expand and stretch a child's experiences.

Play is the best way of introducing ideas about health to the pre-school child. It is possible to introduce basic health concepts through puzzles, stories, songs, acting games, drawing and a range of games (see Figure 9.3).

The school-aged child

There are over a thousand million children of school age in the world. In recent years the developing countries have made great strides in increasing the numbers of children enrolled in primary and secondary schools. In developing countries about 80% of children now enrol in primary or elementary school (ages 6–14).

Why are schools important for health?

Schools can create an educated population who are then better able to make use of the health education they receive in later life from sources such as newspapers, radio and leaflets. This is particularly important in the education of women. Many studies have shown that an educated woman is more likely to take steps to improve the health and nutrition of herself and her family.

It can be difficult for health educators to reach adults directly. Only some adults may visit the clinics and health centres. Mass media such as radio are only suitable for simple messages. Schools provide a way of eventually reaching the whole of a population at an early age before adult behaviours such as diet and smoking are established.

Schools can also directly influence the health of the school child through preventive health measures such as immunisation and dental health as well as screening programmes for early detection of problems in growth and development. In recognition of the importance of schools, in 1995 WHO launched a 'Global School Initiative' which called on governments to take action to promote the spread of 'Health-

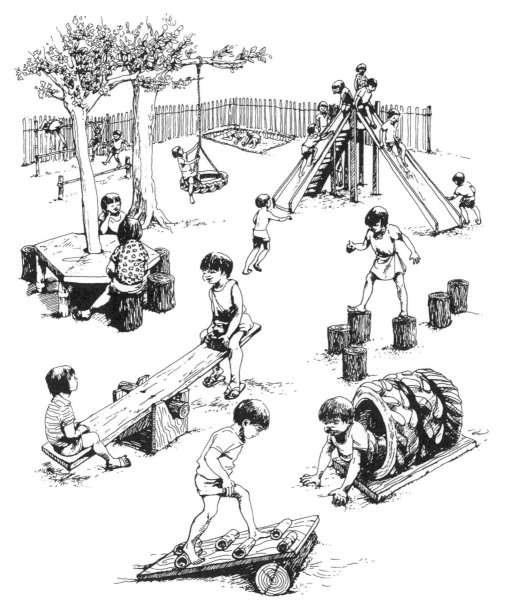

Fig. 9.3 Play and health

Promoting Schools'. According to WHO, a Health-Promoting School:

- strives to improve the health of school personnel, families and community members as well as pupils; and works with community leaders to help them understand how the community contributes to, or undermines, health and education;

- fosters health and learning with all the measures at its disposal;
- strives to provide a healthy environment, school health education, and school health services along with school/community projects and outreach, health promotion programmes for staff, nutrition and food safety programmes, opportunities for physical education and recreation, and programmes for

counselling, social support and mental health promotion;

- implements policies and practices that respect an individual's well-being and dignity, provides multiple opportunities for success, and acknowledges good efforts and intentions as well as personal achievements;
- engages health and education officials, teachers, teachers' unions, students, parents, health providers and community leaders in efforts to make the school a healthy place.

In summary, a school health programme has three components: these are *school health services*; a *health-promoting school environment* and a *school health education programme*. These three components are reinforced by external influences such as support from parents, public education and the primary health care services (see Figure 9.4).

School health services

Depending on local needs and available resources schools can be used for a wide range of important activities that include:

- screening for growth (weight and height), hearing and eyesight;
- immunisations against common childhood diseases including measles and rubella;
- simple preventive and curative treatment for childhood diseases including roundworms, malaria, schistosomiasis, vitamin A deficiency;

- screening for dental health, simple preventive dental services;
- identification of hygiene problems and necessary action, e.g. head-lice infestation;
- counselling for children (and parents) with psychosocial problems affecting their mental health;
- first aid for minor accidents and referral to health services.

Where health workers are scarce, alternatives to doctors and nurses are needed for school health services. Teachers are in close contact with pupils and are in an excellent position to promote health activities.

The school environment

The environment of the school is important for the health of the schoolchild. It also forms part of the 'hidden curriculum' of the school. If schools do not have good provisions for sanitation, clean water and facilities for hygienic preparation of food, children cannot be expected to take seriously the health education they receive in the classroom.

Clean, safe water is needed both for drinking and the washing of hands. The school environment should be kept clean with bins and pits provided for rubbish. Classrooms must be clean and dry with adequate lighting and ventilation.

School meals can have an important role in the nutrition of the schoolchild and many

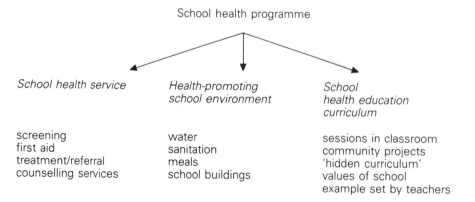

Fig. 9.4   Components of school health programme

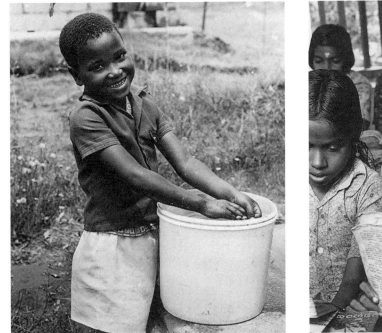
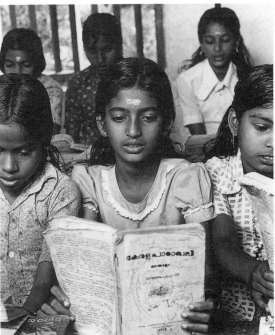
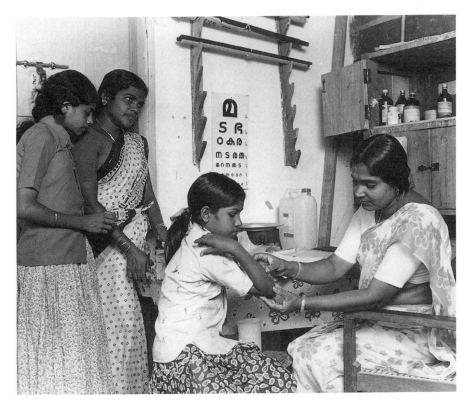

Fig. 9.5   Using schools to improve health

countries have set up feeding programmes. Food should be prepared in clean conditions by properly supervised cooks.

Sanitation is essential for health. Schools should have latrines that must be clean and properly maintained.

Case studies of programmes to strengthen school health services and school environments

Promotion of latrines in the foothills of the Himalayas in East Nepal. Four hundred
secondary school students were trained to build pit latrines in their villages. The schools built demonstration latrines in village markets and used home-made posters and leaflets to persuade villagers to build latrines at their homes. At the end of the pilot phase of the project certificates were given to all families having a pit latrine and a cash prize was awarded to the family with the highest score on the evaluation questionnaire. At the end of the 4-week building period there were 195 pit latrines completed or under construction.

Malaria control through primary schools in Kilifi District of Kenya. Participating schools received a
session that included a drama about malaria and the benefits of insecticide-impregnated mosquito nets. Activities that pupils could do included a poster competition and a survey form to take home. A follow-up visit reinforced the message, discussed the results of the home survey and awarded prizes for the poster competition. A total of 2040 children were reached and an evaluation showed increases in knowledge of malaria. Of the children 54% (1105) had nets at home.

Schistomiasis control through primary schools in Egypt. A 1-day training course was held for
teachers who then provided pupils with health education consisting of modules presented over 3 days, covering the risks from contaminated water, the life cycle of schistosomiasis and the nature and importance of preventive health behaviours including the importance of screening. The methods used included health talks, stories, case histories, role-plays and drama. Evaluation showed that there was a significant improvement in knowledge and attitudes as well as a reduction of schistosomal

infection 1 year after the programme in two of three schools studied, compared with comparison schools which did not receive the intervention.

The 'Health through Sanitation and Water' project (HESAWA) in Tanzania. Between 20 and
30 senior pupils visited each home in the village to collect basic information on the current state of latrines, refuse pits and drying racks. Health workers and teachers then screened school children for nutritional status, intestinal worms and haemoglobin. The village chairman invited parents to a meeting at which they were given a written report on their children's health and were involved in discussing the problems, causes and solutions. An evaluation indicated that villages with HESAWA schools had performed better than other villages in the construction of latrines, dish racks and refuse pits.

Promotion of latrines in Barisal District of rural Bangladesh. A 1-day orientation meeting for local
organisations was followed up by 'courtyard meetings' in communities, and with financial incentives for schools to use pupils to motivate families to build latrines. Attempts were made to involve the local high schools, religious schools, religious leaders and other local leaders in sanitation activities. The District Commissioner announced that the school which achieved the highest sanitation coverage would be rewarded with a contribution towards its development fund. Almost all (91%) of those who had built latrines during the period of the programme reported that they had received communications about latrines from school pupils.

Rheumatic fever in Caribbean islands Martinique and Guadeloupe. A 30-minute film
was shown to teachers, parents and pupils in schools. Pamphlets describing the clinical features and origin of cardiac complications of rheumatic fever were distributed to school children's parents and patients attending hospital clinics. Posters were placed in schools and hospitals and supporting messages were broadcast on radio and television. The first months of the programme led to a 10–20% increase in the number of people coming to hospital with rheumatic fever. During the life of the programme there was a decline in prevalence of rheumatic fever.

The school health education programme

Timetabled lessons and projects in health education

In many countries only a small proportion of children go on to secondary school. So, to reach everyone, there should be a planned comprehensive curriculum with timetabled sessions in health education starting from the first year of primary school and extending up to secondary school. These sessions can include classroom activities and practical activities in the community such as making a survey of local water supplies.

The Child-to-Child programme encourages children to undertake community projects (see description below). Older children can be selected as 'health guides' and are then involved in teaching younger pupils. This powerful health education technique is called peer teaching and relies for effectiveness on the fact that younger pupils often have great respect and try to copy older pupils. Sometimes they listen to the older pupils more than they do their teachers!

Health education as part of other subjects

It is often difficult to find space in the timetable for health education. There may be pressure to emphasise the 'core curriculum' subjects such as Mathematics, English and Science that are important for gaining a place in secondary school. A challenging solution to this problem is to build health issues into other subjects. Obvious subjects for including health issues are Home Economics, Biology, Environmental Studies, Physical Education and Agriculture.

However, there are other less obvious subjects that can be used for health education. Local language and English language classes can be used for reading and writing about health. English has a high priority in the 'core' curriculum in many counties. The *Living Health* project is a series of graded English language readers published by Macmillan, which contain stories with a health focus (e.g. AIDS, latrines, malaria, first aid) together with a fact file with information about the topic and activities for the reader.

Art can be used for painting on health issues, Music for health songs, Drama to show health topics and Religious Education for discussions of values and relationships.

Mathematics provides many opportunities for considering health. A workshop held in Kenya by Child-to-Child has produced a book describing how health examples can be used to teach many basic mathematical concepts including shapes, numbers, graphs, measurement and fractions. Practical activities include counting malaria breeding sites, numbers of children and the elderly. 'Child health charts' provide a way to introduce graphs and weights while also discussing an extremely important topic in child health (charts are available from TALC – see Appendix). Oral rehydration of children with diarrhoea could form the basis for a science lesson on water and salts.

Out-of-school activities

Many schools have clubs and other out-of-school activities where health topics can be covered. For example, societies such as the Red Cross, Red Crescent, Boy Scouts and Girl Guides provide opportunities for learning about first aid and other health topics. In some countries in Africa, anti-AIDS clubs have been set up where children learn about AIDS and how to prevent it. An advantage of out-of-school settings is that is possible to be more relaxed and informal.

The hidden curriculum

The hidden curriculum of the school environment and the teachers' behaviours are important influences and have already been discussed. What children are taught in the classroom should be practised by the teachers!

Learning methods for school health education

Many people have been critical of traditional teaching approaches in schools that overemphasise learning facts and passing exams. In health education we usually want to do more than give children facts. We wish to equip them to make decisions, explore attitudes and values and adopt healthy practices both now and in their future lives. Summarised here are the approaches that are increasingly being emphasised in school health education; some examples of school-based health education activities are described in the Case studies on pages 175–177.

Recent approaches in school health education

Child-centred approach – placing the emphasis on meeting the needs of the children, starting with the child's perception of a healthy lifestyle and recognising that children learn at different rates. The ideas introduced at each level of primary and secondary schooling should reflect the social/emotional, physical and intellectual development of the child.

Active learning methods that encourage exploration and discovery and relate the information presented to everyday life – bridging the gap between home and community.

Problem-solving or 'issue-based' learning which organises the learning around issues or problems rather than traditional subject disciplines. In this approach, students usually take a health topic and carry out a range of activities in the classroom, at home and in the community. Their finished project might include: songs, drawing, arithmetic, science experiments and story writing.

Decision-making methods – role-plays and exercises where children learn to take decisions. This might include role-play where a young person has opportunities to try out different responses to another person's attempt to persuade them to smoke a cigarette, take alcohol or have sex.

Life-skills – methods which promote decision-making and use a variety of active learning methods, such as role-play and case studies, to help young people face the challenges that they meet now and in their future life.

Peer teaching methods – which encourage the use of older respected children as 'peer models'. For example an older child might tell younger children that it is not particularly grown up to smoke cigarettes.

Self-esteem enhancement – this involves educational approaches that make children develop confidence in themselves and their worth and reduce feelings of failure; children with high self-esteem are more likely to have the confidence to resist pressure from others to engage in risky behaviour.

Teacher-based approaches rather than relying on external visitors – teachers are in the school all the time and know the children better than visitors. Emphasis should be placed on using the teachers themselves as much as possible rather than external visitors to do the health education.

Health education in primary and secondary schools

The most important task in developing a curriculum is to plan the content to match the level and age of the child as she/he progresses through the school. This involves taking into account the various stages of social/emotional, intellectual and physical development that are discussed earlier in the chapter. The primary school is a good time for laying the foundations of health that can be built upon in later schooling. However, in early primary school the child can only grasp simple concepts and ideas. Only later will a child be able to handle more complex and abstract arguments. The spread of content across the different ages may have to be modified for another practical reason. In many countries only a few of children go on to secondary school. This means that the health education in the primary school must aim to be as comprehensive as possible to prepare the child for future life.

The secondary school provides an opportunity to build upon the foundations laid by the school health education in the primary school. However, some special problems face health education in secondary schools. Health education may not have been covered well in the primary school so there is no foundation of learning about health to build upon in the secondary school. Emphasis on academic subjects and examinations may restrict time on 'non-essential' subjects like health education. Often health education is carried out in a 'crisis oriented' approach with visiting speakers brought in to tell pupils of the 'dangers' of alcohol, drugs, tobacco, sex and AIDS. These sessions are not integrated within a broad-based health education programme.

Special problems can be encountered with sex education. Community leaders and parents may not approve of sex education in schools. Teachers can be unwilling to deal with subjects they find embarrassing. There is plenty of evidence of the need for sex education among schoolchildren: a survey of more than 100 Kenyan schoolgirls who became pregnant showed that 65 had never received any information about contraception; studies of how young people learn about sex show that young people often pick up most of their knowledge about fertility and contraception from friends and the media – and much of this is incomplete, misleading and wrong. Myths and misconceptions are common – for example many young people mistakenly believe that pregnancy cannot occur if they are very young, they are having sex for the first time or do not have intercourse very often. Also many are mistaken about when the fertile part of the menstrual cycle occurs. Many countries were reluctant to include sex education in their curriculum but have now changed their policy because of the risk of AIDS.

Recent approaches to health education in secondary school children have emphasised a move away from crisis-oriented approaches towards a *planned curriculum* that builds on a foundation laid in primary school. Health Education is linked with other developments including counselling, career advisory services and social education. Sex should not be dealt with in isolation. It should be part of a wider *'family life education'* emphasising responsible relationships, plans for career, preparation for future roles as parents, development of self-esteem and an examination of the pressures from family, friends and society to act in particular ways. With teenage pupils it is best to use the participatory learning approaches described in Chapter 4. For example, young girls can role-play being asked by a boy to have sex and explore different ways they could respond. Boys can role-play being a girl and becoming pregnant and thus develop understandings of responsible behaviour. A family life education curriculum could consist of the following:

- family structures, roles and responsibilities;
- growing to maturity including sexual development;
- self-awareness, decision-making and forming relationships;
- parenthood, antenatal care, childbirth, child care;
- biology of sexual intercourse, conception and childbirth;
- methods of contraception; and
- population changes in society.

Case studies of health education programmes in schools

Mental health promotion programme in Rawalpindi, Pakistan. Training in mental health promotion was given to secondary school teachers. Teachers went on to introduce an educational programme which included introduction of participatory teaching methods and other activities including inputs at annual speech days, drama productions, essay-writing and poster-painting competitions and involvement of parent–teacher associations. An evaluation in two schools showed that the programme had achieved an increase in awareness of mental health issues and a reduction in stigma and prejudice towards persons who were mentally ill.

Sex education in Caribbean Islands of St Kitts and Nevis. A syllabus covering human reproduction, growth and development, emotional development and issues and values in adolescent sexuality was developed for the 12–15 age group to be delivered through two 40-minute sessions. A follow-up evaluation at 10–12 months found an impact on knowledge but no effect on sexual practices or use of contraception when compared with schools not receiving the programme.

Eye health promotion in a middle school in Harayana, India. Eight pupils were given intensive training on eye health including vitamin A, trachoma, injury prevention (e.g. from ball games, bows and arrows and fireworks) and refractive errors. Teachers were also briefed and materials provided. One week later each of the 'child health educators' spoke to the rest of their school for 3 minutes on a topic. At the end of the session doctors summarised points. An evaluation found that there was an improvement in knowledge of symptoms of trachoma, risks of eye injuries and sources of vitamin A.

Blindness prevention in Metahara town, Ethiopia. Primary school children were given a multiple-choice test followed by explanations and discussions. They were then given the assignment of writing a story and drawing pictures about two families where one does everything wrong and some of its members become blind; the other does everything right and all of its members have healthy eyes. Knowledge about prevention of blindness increased; there were fewer children with dirty faces and prevalence of trachoma and conjunctivitis decreased over the following year.

The First AIDS Kit for teenagers in schools in South Africa. The First AIDS Kit was an AIDS and lifestyle education programme for teenagers. The programme was based around the Theory of Reasoned Action, The Health Belief Model and the self-efficacy approach. The kit consisted of five modules covering: (1) adolescence; (2) AIDS and STDs; (3) relationships; (4) life skills; and (5) safe sex skills. The kit included a video, a quiz to teach facts, and exercises in assertiveness, decision-making, negotiation skills and choosing low-risk behaviours. Teachers were encouraged to select parts of the kit that they considered appropriate to the students' needs. An evaluation found improvements in knowledge but no change in behavioural intention and perception of condom use.

AIDS education in secondary schools in Malawi. A team from the University of Malawi developed and introduced a board game 'The AIDS Challenge'. A group of 72 pupils aged 13–20 were selected from one school. These students were given a questionnaire and then played the game weekly for 4 weeks. Their test score increased each time the game was played and the improvements were sustained when the test was re-administered a month later.

AIDS education for Zulu-speaking high school pupils in South Africa. A play about AIDS was presented to students who were then given the opportunity to attend drama workshops to design their own plays, songs and poetry. These were presented at an open day. A self-completed questionnaire was given to 72 Zulu-speaking high school pupils from each participating class before and after drama intervention. Mean knowledge scores increased and there was a decrease in the number of pupils who agreed with the statement 'I would like to have more than one sexual partner'.

Sex education for secondary school pupils from 11 rural schools in Zimbabwe. Classroom sessions supported by videos, leaflets, pamphlets and posters were given on reproductive biology, STD/HIV/AIDS, unwanted pregnancy, contraception, human sexuality and responsible behaviour. An evaluation found a significant increase in correct knowledge about aspects of menstruation in intervention schools as compared with controls. Knowledge about wet dreams increased. Pupils from intervention schools were more likely to know that a boy aged between 13–19 years could make a girl pregnant and that a girl could get pregnant at her first sexual intercourse.

An AIDS education programme among high school students in Manila, Philippines. Thirty teachers attended a 2-day workshop on AIDS education and a core group of participating teachers were involved in the design of a school-based educational curriculum. The curriculum covered five areas: human sexuality and STDs, AIDS, the immune system, development of self-esteem, decision-making skills and refusal skills. The educational programme consisted of 12 lessons taught as two 40-minute lessons per week over 6 weeks. As well as traditional lectures, sessions included role-playing, games, dialogues, group discussions and exercises. Support materials included a teacher's manual, flip charts and audiotapes. An evaluation showed that, compared with a group of schools that did not receive the education, in intervention schools pupils receiving the education had higher levels of HIV-related knowledge and scored higher positive attitudes (less likely to avoid people with AIDS and more likely to show compassion to persons with AIDS).

Schistosomiasis control in primary schools Dongting Lakes Region, China. After initial research an intervention programme was developed to increase children's knowledge of schistosomiasis as an environmental disease and to encourage them to reduce their contact with unsafe water sources. Pupils were shown a video followed by 10 minutes of discussion and received a comic book. The video used a cartoon format to tell the story of a group of children who did not know where the 'demons' (i.e. schistosomes) hid in their environment. An angel – representing a health worker – told the children which places were safe and which were unsafe. A song ran through the programme reinforcing the message. After the intervention, knowledge about schistosomiasis was much higher and use of unsafe water sites was less in the intervention group compared with a group of children who were not exposed to the programme.

Dental health education programme in primary schools in Tanzania. A training course was provided for teachers who then taught sessions on oral health and care of teeth using the activity-based methods that they had learnt. When compared with schools receiving no oral health education, pupils in the schools that received modified oral health education had better knowledge of oral health, reported reduced consumption of sugary foods and increased self-reported tooth brushing frequency, had better *mswaki* (chewing stick) making skills and slightly improved oral hygiene.

The Child-to-Child Programme

The International Year of the Child in 1979 saw the launching of the Child-to-Child programme which has since expanded to more than 70 countries in the world. According to Hugh Hawes, one of the founders, the Child-to-Child programme is based on three fundamental assumptions:

1 that primary education becomes more effective if it is linked closely to things that matter most to children and to their families and communities;
2 that education in school and education out of school should be linked as closely as possible so that learning becomes a part of life;

3 that children have the will, the skill and the motivation to help educate each other and can be trusted to do so.

In its early stages, the Child-to-Child programme placed special emphasis on the idea of using the primary school child to reach out to younger brothers and sisters. The approach has now widened to include a wide range of new and exciting approaches for promotion of health in schools.

Eleven key messages were originally identified and these are shown in Table 9.1. Each message is accompanied by a series of practical activities that would be realistic, interesting and fun for children to undertake. Activity sheets (which are distributed free from the address in the Appendix) were prepared (see Figure 9.6). These encouraged children to:

• identify an issue that is a local priority and find out about the health topic;

Table 9.1 Key messages in Child-to-Child Programme

Personal and community hygiene and safety	Prevent accidents. Care for teeth. Promote neighbourhood hygiene.
Prevention and control of disease	Oral rehydration saves the lives of children with diarrhoea. Learn to recognise danger signs of illness. Care for sick children.
Child stimulation and development	Play and mental stimulation help children develop. Toys and games can be made that aid growth and development.
Recognising and helping those with disabilities	Children with sight and hearing problems need to be identified and their prob lems understood. Signs of malnutrition can be recognised and its causes understood. Better feeding is usually possible even through more money may not be available.

Child-to-Child

Activity Sheet 4.1

Child-to-Child Activity Sheets are a resource for teachers, and health and community workers. They are designed to help children understand how to improve health in other children, their families, and their communities. Topics chosen are important for community health and suit the age, interests and experience of children. The text, ideas and activities may be freely adapted to suit local conditions.

PREVENTING ACCIDENTS

THE IDEA

In some places, as many as two children in a school die each year because of accidents. Many more will be injured. **These accidents need not happen.** Children can help to reduce the number and seriousness of accidents by practising safety at home, out-of-doors and on the road. Children can learn to spot the most common dangers, and understand how these dangers can be avoided or prevented. They should always watch out for the safety of others, particularly smaller children.

Children can also be prepared to help when an accident happens.

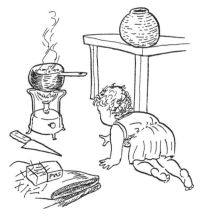

Children can talk about the accidents which they have seen happen most often in their community. Different sorts of accidents happen to children who live in different places - in towns, in villages, in rural areas. Identify accidents which have happened in the last six months at home, on the road, anywhere out-of-doors and discuss **why** they happened.

At Home

- **burns** from cooking pots or lamps, electrical appliances, hot food, boiling water, steam, hot fat (scalds), strong acid or corrosives (like battery acid) which damage the skin;
- **cuts** from broken glass, rusty pins, rough wood or sharp knives and axes;
- **obstruction (preventing) of breathing** from swallowing small objects like coins, buttons and nuts;
- **poisoning** from eating or drinking harmful things;
- **internal (inside) bleeding** from swallowing sharp objects like razor blades;
- **electric shock** from touching a broken electrical appliance or electrical wire.

On the Road

- **death** or injuries like heavy **bleeding, broken bones** and **damage to main organs** of the body (liver, lungs, brain) (*see* Sheet 4.2, Road Safety).

In the Playground or Out-of-Doors

- **burns, cuts** and **broken bones**;
- **poisoning** from eating certain plants and berries;
- **bites** from animals and snakes and stings from bees and other insects;
- **drowning** in open water or wells.

This sheet can be used together with Sheet No. 4.2, **Road** Safety and Sheet No. 4.3, **First Aid.**

Fig. 9.6   A Child-to-Child worksheet

- gather information on the extent and nature of health topic in the home and community;
- organise and discuss findings and plan action;
- take action in the school, community or home to tackle the problem;
- evaluate the impact of the actions – discuss the results;
- discuss how to be more effective next time.

A survey carried out of 114 Child-to-Child Projects in 39 countries showed that activities undertaken fell into three broad groups. The largest single group of activities were *'outreach projects'* where children applied their knowledge to help others in the community. For example a report from Kenya described how the head-master, teachers and pupils of a primary school worked with the children at a school in their community for children with disabilities. They made crutches for children with some physical disabilities. The primary school children and the children with disabilities enjoyed working and learning together.

The next largest single group were *'enquiry projects'* (28%) where children used Child-to-Child materials and investigations to acquire knowledge that they will use later. One report from Fiji described how 'As a schoolteacher I and my colleagues have used Child-to-Child materials in health education to advance children's knowledge through reading and through activity. The children were involved in carrying out experiments and in collecting data and other records. Since these activities are child-oriented it gives them a chance for self-discovery.'

The third group consisted of a mixture of approaches where the Child-to-Child materials were used in the classroom and for training of teachers. In another review of Child-to-Child

---

Some 'Child-to-Child' methods for school health education

Chalk and talk: using the chalkboard; making lists, e.g. foods at market; classifying information; prepare action plans, e.g. for a clean-up programme; write out instructions; measuring things and summarising information on graph or chart.

Picture talks: drawing pictures on chalkboard, on paper; cutting out pictures for flannelgraphs, flipcharts, comic books; story rolls; asking questions about each picture; making a mural (large wall painting).

Storytelling: telling stories at class, school assemblies, while waiting at health centres; telling stories to younger children; making pictures to accompany stories; putting pictures in flip charts and flannelgraphs.

Songs: making up songs about health topics.

Dramatisations: acting out stories; dressing up and performing plays; use role-play to imagine what It is like being in a situation; make and perform puppet plays to other children and the community.

Reading and writing: reading health stories; comics, newspapers. magazines, posters and pamphlets; writing health stories and messages; writing letters about local activities; making health posters; making record cards; preparing school newspapers and notice boards.

Experiments and demonstrations: making, doing, growing, weighing, measuring things; observing things, discussing them, tell others about them, portraying them in dramas, plays, puppet shows or exhibitions.

Projects and campaigns: in the school and community.

Table 9.2 Example of integrated project approach

Topic: children should be able to establish the relationship between polluted water and disease.	
SUBJECT AREAS	**ACTIVITIES and TEACHING METHODS**
Oral expression	Telling about the sickness. Question children about their opinion
Educational games	Sequence of pictures and/or comic strips about the different phases of diarrhoea: a child drinks polluted water, has stomach pains, has diarrhoea
Visits	Go to the health centre, question the nurse
Mathematical activity	Ask children about diarrhoea among their younger brothers and sisters. Plot the results on a histogram to show how common it is
Graphics	Ask children to draw pictures of themselves when sick
Symbolic games (drama)	Mime sickness in a simple play. Make puppets and prepare a show. Play a scene about the disease and how to treat it with oral rehydration solution
Songs and stories	Make up a song about water and health
Reading	Read story from Child-to-Child reader about dirty water
Science	Discuss nature of water, salts and sugars
Practical activity	Make oral rehydration solution up for a child with diarrhoea

programmes, Audrey Aarons suggested the active learning methods listed here. An example of a project-based activity is also given in Table 9.2.

Setting up a school health programme

A starting point is for health workers, parents and teachers to meet and discuss their common interests and needs. Health education is usually in the school syllabus but may not be taught well or given much priority. Parents often want their children to do well at school and gain academic qualifications and can resist any move away from traditional academic subjects. However you can use the argument that a healthy child performs better at school to persuade education authorities, teachers and parents to support the expansion of health-promoting activities.

From these discussions you can develop a policy for developing a school health programme covering each of the three areas described above of school health services, school environment and health education. Some of the questions you will have to ask to develop your curriculum are listed below.

Questions to ask when planning a school health programme.

- What do parents, teachers, pupils, community leaders and health workers feel about the need to expand health education in schools? What topics do they feel should be a priority? How do they feel about each topic area including sensitive subjects such as sex education?
- Is there already a health education curriculum? How much scope for improvement is there through teacher training, improved resources within the present curriculum? Does the curriculum have to be changed? Can this be done locally or is the curriculum determined at the national level?
- How should the content be organised to ensure an integrated comprehensive curriculum rather

than a crisis-oriented approach? How much time should be allocated to timetabled sessions on health education? How much emphasis should be placed on expanding health education within existing subjects such as Mathematics, English and Science? How can the curriculum be organised in each school year to meet the child's changing physical, social/emotional and intellectual development as well as health needs? Should health education be assessed in examinations? How can the curriculum reflect the needs of the community and the national culture?

- Do existing teaching methods in the schools need to be changed to allow effective school health education? What scope is there for project-based activities, field visits and 'Child-to-Child' activities?
- What preparation do teachers need to undertake school health education? How should this training be organised? What support do they need, such as educational materials, and how can these be provided?
- What scope is there for expanding out-of-school activities such as clubs and sports to support the school health programme?
- What improvement in the school infrastructure of water supply, toilets, waste disposal, school meals are needed to support the educational activities?
- What organisational structure, such as a school health committee, is needed to bring together interested groups such as health workers, parents and teachers to plan and implement school health promotion activities?

A good example of a national curriculum development approach is the school health education programme in Uganda. A national committee was set up with representatives from the Ministry of Health, Ministry of Education and other interested groups. It was decided to locate the health education within the existing science curriculum and make it an examinable subject. The curriculum was tested in 20 schools and covers topics such as nutrition, safe water, sanitation, immunisation, the treatment of common diseases, the prevention of accidents and AIDS. A series of 'training of trainers' workshops was held to create a network of trainers. These trainers went on to run workshops for teachers in every district on how to implement the new curriculum. With the assistance of UNICEF, sets of attractive support materials were produced including wallcharts and a teachers' guide.

Some people criticise centralised curriculum development approaches because they do not always meet needs of local communities. They also represent a 'top-down' approach and miss out on the opportunities presented when teachers, parents and health workers work together to develop school health programmes. In a district-based approach to curriculum development in the South Indian State of Kerala, one teacher was selected from each of 30 schools to be a health education coordinator. They were responsible for development of the school health programme in their school, coordination of health education activities and supporting the health education activities of other teachers. The teachers were trained on: simple treatment and prevention of local diseases; first aid; and a range of health education activities including project-based health education approaches. On return to their schools they set up school health committees, attended sick children, started screening activities and set up a variety of school health education activities in the school and community.

If you cannot work at the national or district level you can still work among the schools in your immediate community. If you have not had much experience of schools it is essential to talk to local teachers and see how they feel about health education and what could be done at the local level. Find out what scope there is for improving the quantity and quality of health promotion activities within the present curriculum. A list of helpful books on school health education and some addresses of resource agencies are given in the Appendix.

Reaching children out-of-school

Out-of-school children include the following groups each with their distinct needs:

- school children in their spare time;

- children who have left school early and are now working, e.g. children of poor landless families in rural areas who are needed for daily activities such as collecting firewood, looking after animals and caring for children;
- children who have never gone to school at all – these could be children orphaned by wars and disease, deserted by their parents through poverty; also important are the growing numbers of 'street children' in cities of Latin America, Africa and Asia who earn money from petty trading, parking cars, and in some situations theft and child prostitution.

When they leave school, young people become more independent from their parents and begin to earn money that they may spend going out to bars and discos. They are more likely to be sexually active than schoolchildren at the same age.

Young people out-of-school are one of the most difficult groups to reach. If they attend youth clubs or church groups, educational activities can be carried out in these informal locations. However, many young people do not attend clubs and special approaches are needed to reach these groups.

Young people in urban areas are often interested in music and have their 'youth culture' with distinctive styles of clothing, hair and music. In Uganda a video was made of a song and drama on AIDS produced by a musician who was looked up to and highly regarded by young people. This approach was also used in the pop record made by 'Tatiana and Johnny' described in the Chapter 7 on popular media. In Swaziland the National AIDS Committee carried out a survey of young people to find out which radio programmes they listened to and used this information to help them decide how best to plan their educational strategy.

The emergence of AIDS has raised many people's concerns about street children – especially because a growing number of them are forced into making a living through child prostitution. An interesting programme in Mexico was sponsored by the organisation Street Kids International. They produced a cartoon film on video that featured a hero character 'Karate Kid' and used it in educational projects with street children

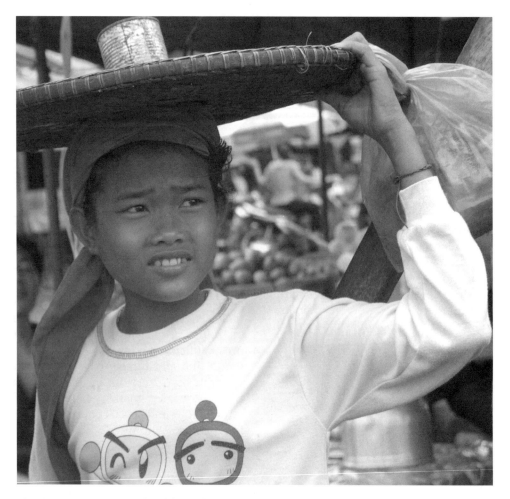

Fig. 9.7   Programmes should reach children who are working

on AIDS (see Figure 9.9). The Copperbelt Health Education Project in Zambia developed an educational programme among street children. They ran a 1-week workshop for street children that included the following sessions: staying healthy (covering AIDS, STDs, drug abuse, alcohol abuse and cigarette smoking and including a visit to the local hospital); staying within the law (including a visit to the local police station); going back to the land (a visit to a farm training centre); running a successful small business (including basic arithmetic and accountancy); and locally available skills training opportunities.

One advantage of educational programmes outside school is that it is possible to be much more informal and relaxed than in school or in the presence of parents. It is a good opportunity to use the participatory learning methods described in Chapter 4 including group discussion, games and role-plays. Young people will want to show independence from their parents and will expect to be taken seriously. Indeed, if they have been able to survive in the difficult environment of a city street, they will know a great deal already about life and resent being talked to like children. Their experiences are a resource to build upon. If their participation is encouraged, they will be able to suggest appropriate methods and strategies for reaching other young people.

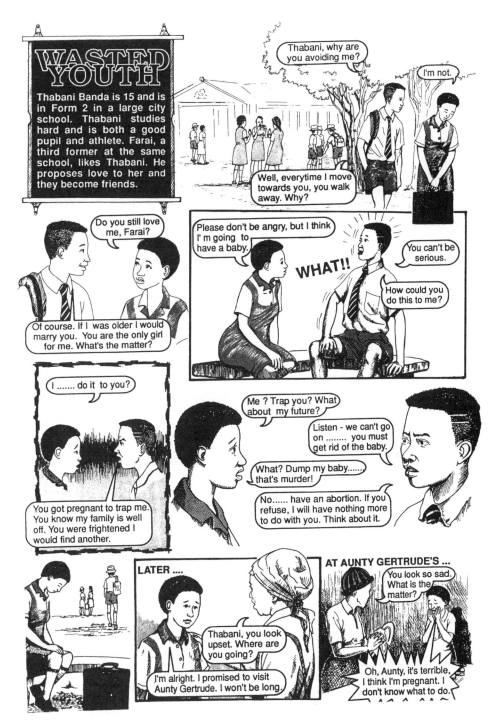

Fig. 9.8   A page from *Action* comic in Zimbabwe

Some promising health education approaches for working with young people are to:

- use people that young people look up to such as singers or football players to speak on health issues;
- ask popular music groups to perform songs about health issues;
- use young people as fieldworkers that youths will listen and respond to;
- involve young people themselves in producing a drama about their lives and situation;
- train a group of young volunteers to carry out informal health education in the bars and discos where the young people go;
- include health issues in the initiation ceremonies that are carried out for both boys and girls in many countries and serve as traditional forms of sex education.

Alongside the attention to health education, increasing attention is being placed on reorienting health services to meet the needs of young people. Young people may be reluctant to use existing health services because they feel that services for adults will not meet their special needs, they are afraid that a judgemental approach will be used by the adults who run them, and they are afraid that information will be passed on to their parents. In response to these concerns, some programmes directed at young people have set up 'youth-friendly' services, which offer a confidential service that is specifically designed to meet the needs of young people and staffed by health workers who are sympathetic to the needs of young persons and trained to be supportive and non-judgemental. Services provided include advice and treatment for a range of health topics (especially reproductive health), counselling, peer education, family planning and general psychosocial support.

Case studies of health promotion activities with young people

Kenya Youth Initiatives Project. The Youth Variety Show was an interactive, hour-long English-language radio programme that was broadcast on Saturday mornings. The show was hosted by well-known personalities and was designed to provide young people with information related to growing up, with a special focus on reproductive health. Each episode featured a panel of adolescents and expert guests who would discuss various issues to stimulate open dialogue. Telephone calls from young listeners were also taken on the air to encourage participation and exchange of perspectives and experiences, and to answer questions. A total of 79 episodes were broadcast. An evaluation found that they had been listened to by 3.3 million adolescents, 800,000 of whom reported that they had taken some form of action as a result of the show, and 60,000 had visited a youth clinic or telephoned or written to the programme producers. The cost amounted to US$ 0.12 per youth reached.

The Soweto Adolescent Reproductive Health Programme in South Africa. A group of 70 Soweto youths were trained in participatory media development, peer education and condom distribution, and 3000 condom distribution outlets were set up. The youths developed materials including radio advertisements, posters, T-shirts, badges, slogans and a 44-page adolescent sexuality booklet. Soweto Community Radio and Voice of Soweto broadcast weekly 2-hour talk shows, which included live phone-in questions and discussions. A six-part documentary on condoms and safer sex was produced for South African TV and for showing as videos. A survey found that among young people in the target community there was increased awareness of the risk of becoming pregnant, that condoms can prevent HIV/AIDS, that young people can take steps to prevent pregnancy, STDs and HIV/AIDS.

Sex education among young men average age 18 years in urban slums in Lucknow, India. Three educational sessions lasting 1 hour each were carried out at 3-week intervals. During the last 15 minutes of each session, a taped set of educational messages about sexual health was played followed by an opportunity for individual counselling if required. A voluntary urine test to detect bacterial infections was provided at the second session to generate information to feed back to the young people at the third session. An evaluation found significant increases in knowledge about symptoms of STDs and also increased awareness that STDs could be caught from women other than sex workers.

The Entre Nous Jeunes peer-educator programme in Nkongsamba town in Cameroon. Over an 18-month period, 42 young persons were recruited from schools and youth associations and given a 1-week training programme. These peer educators worked as volunteers leading 353 discussion groups, one-on-one meetings and sessions at health and sports associations. Promotional materials including calendars, comic strips, posters, T-shirts, baseball caps and bags were distributed to 5000 adolescents. An evaluation found that young people who had had contact with peer educators had greater knowledge of STDs and were more likely to be using contraception, including condoms.

The Young People's Project in the Philippines. A multimedia campaign centred around two pop songs and music videos with messages about sexual responsibility and prevention of teenage pregnancy. These coincided with the launching of a telephone hotline 'Dial-a-friend' using volunteer counsellors. The song hit top of the charts in several radio stations and received high coverage in newspapers and television. An evaluation found that most young people could recall the song and understood it. Almost half the sample had talked about their sexual behaviour with friends and a quarter said that they had sought information about contraceptives as a result of hearing about the programme.

Mass media campaign to reach young people in St Lucia, St Vincent and the Grenadines and Grenada, Eastern Caribbean. A radio campaign lasting 2 months was targeted primarily at parents of teenage children. The central message was 'When you can't protect them any more … condoms can'. Parents were urged to talk to their teenagers about sexual responsibility and safer sex. A follow-up survey found that young people exposed to the message were significantly more likely: to believe that it is possible to protect

oneself from AIDS; to believe that parents and teens should discuss sexual responsibility; and to be aware of the existence of the AIDS hotline. The campaign did not appear to increase the level of condom use.

Summary

There is enormous scope for expanding and improving health education activities for pre-school children, schoolchildren and out-of-school youth and if you wish to take this further you can consult the list of reading and addresses provided in the Appendix. It is possible to draw the following general conclusions.

- There is a need to expand the quantity and quality of educational interventions directed at young children. Special efforts are needed to meet the needs of those groups in society with the worst health: usually the poorest; children of parents with few educational qualifications; children who have missed out on school; and girls.
- Health education should bridge the gap between school and community through relevant content, community projects and involvement of parents and community leaders; the curriculum should consider health problems in the community and the influence of the family, friends and community.
- Educational methods should match the developmental stage of the child; they should go beyond just giving facts and be action-oriented and enquiry-based; and develop thinking ability and decision-making. Teachers will need training and support to enable them to introduce these methods.
- School-based programmes should be supported by other interventions to reach those children not attending school.
- Educational programmes directed at children should be part of a comprehensive community-based primary health care approach with the full participation of health workers, teachers, parents, pupils and the community.

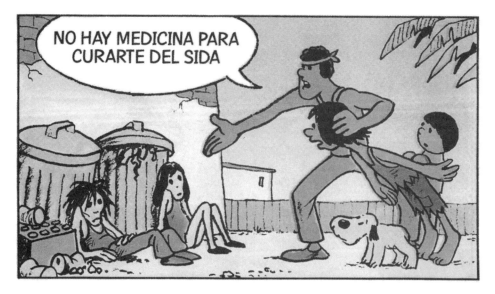

Fig. 9.9   The Karate Kid in Mexico – 'There is no medicine to cure AIDS'

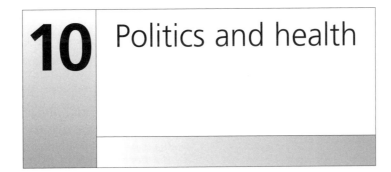

10 Politics and health

In looking at health problems and their causes we have seen that there are limits to what can be achieved by working at the individual level. In particular, I have emphasised the danger of *victim blaming* – where we focus our educational activities on the individual and ignore external factors such as pressure from others, poverty, lack of facilities and opportunities for change. It is not enough just to help people make decisions. We have to make it easier for them to make healthy choices.

In the list below are just a few of the political, social and economic factors that can influence health and make healthy choices. These include government policies concerning:

- military expenditure and war;
- human rights;
- actions that increase poverty, social inequalities and unemployment;
- policies affecting the status of women and children;
- policies leading to harmful environmental changes, e.g. deforestation, pesticides, dumping of toxic wastes, release of carbon dioxide and other 'greenhouse' gases;
- policies affecting urbanisation, availability of adequate housing, water and sanitation;
- costs of foods, subsidies for agriculture, imports;
- pricing and availability of basic commodities such as foods, clothing, soap, transport;
- laws to remove hazards from the workplace;
- pricing of harmful substances such as tobacco, alcohol and baby milk substitutes;
- advertising of health-damaging products;
- actions by multinational companies;
- spending on health care and education;
- accessibility and appropriateness of health care services and commitment to primary health care.

Most of these topics take us outside the traditional work of health services. As individuals, we often feel helpless when faced with the immense task of trying to influence our own government or other countries. Yet these factors are crucial to the creation of a healthy society. If we take seriously our task of promoting health, we cannot simply walk away from these responsibilities and say that they are not our concern.

It was in response to these concerns that many people became dissatisfied with the traditional view of health education that put too much emphasis on the individual and not enough on community action and government action. In Chapter 1 of this book, I described the broader concept of *health promotion* that includes health education as well as advocacy to influence government policies that concern health.

Some of the different ways in which communities can come together to work for change were described in Chapter 6. In particular, I discussed how the ideas of Paulo Freire could be applied to develop the critical awareness of disadvantaged groups and their ability to challenge and change their surroundings. The use of drama for raising consciousness and stimulating social action was described in the Chapter 7. This chapter will look at examples of how individuals and groups have managed to influence governments, and work at the national and international level for political and social action.

Nutrition and food security

Food security exists when all people at all times, have physical, social and economic access to sufficient, safe and nutritious food to meet their dietary needs and food preferences for an active and healthy life. Household food security is the application of this concept at the family level, with individuals within households as the focus of concern.

United Nations Food and Agriculture Organization (FAO)

The FAO estimates that more than 800 million people in the world are undernourished and that most of these are in the developing world. In the past, nutrition education has tended to emphasise the individual person and his or her choice of food. However, as shown in Figure 10.1, the individual is really at the end of a series of stages from cultivation, marketing, purchasing, food processing and sharing out in the home. The actual food received by a member of a family is the result of many different factors, only some of which are under a person's control. Some factors such as food availability, income and women's time are seasonal and change during the year.

According to FAO, food insecurity is a result of factors which include:

- *the socio-economic and political environment* – economy, agriculture, education, natural resources, population;
- *the performance of the food economy* – food production, imports, prices, incomes, markets;
- *care practices* including child care, feeding practices, food preparation, eating habits and distribution of food in the home;
- *health and sanitation* – water quality, hygiene practices, sanitation and health care practices.

Nutrition and food consumption are influenced by national policies. Most important of these are the prices paid to farmers and whether incentives are given to plant particular crops. For example, cash crops may be encouraged rather than food crops. In the colonial period many countries such as Ghana, Kenya and Mauritius were encouraged to devote their best land to cash crops for the colonial power and this pattern continued after independence. Attempts to

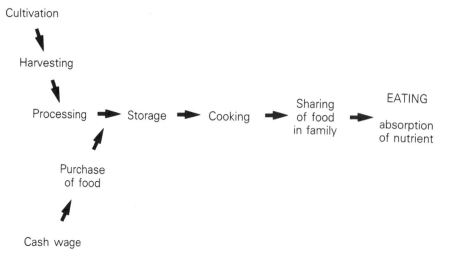

Fig. 10.1 The food pathway

transfer more land to cultivation of food have been made difficult by the need to obtain foreign exchange to pay back debts to the West and the fall in prices of cash crops. Furthermore, cash crops can themselves be health-damaging as you will see when the issue of smoking and tobacco control is discussed later in the chapter.

Measures that increase agricultural productivity can have harmful effects on health. The overuse of pesticides is affecting the ecological balance by killing beneficial insects as well as pests. It also can directly harm health through accidental poisoning of agricultural workers and entry of pesticides into the foods we eat. Large-scale irrigation projects have had some unexpected side effects. These include providing breeding sites for malaria mosquitoes and the snails that spread schistosomiasis.

The importing, marketing and advertising of foods can have implications for health. In West Africa, locally produced palm oil is rich in vitamin A and, unlike imported cooking oil, prevents blindness from vitamin A deficiency. Imports of cooking oil have led to reduced production of palm oil. Consumer products, e.g. drinking chocolate, are heavily advertised and promoted as modern. Many processed foods are not directly harmful (although as you will see later in this chapter baby milk substitutes are definitely harmful). However, they encourage people to spend money on expensive prestige products when the same money could buy a substantial amount of locally-produced nutritious food.

Agriculturalists and economists dealing with pricing and import controls rarely take health and nutrition issues into account. Yet their decisions have a profound effect on health. A challenge for health educators is to learn to work more closely with these groups to develop food policies that promote health.

Intersectoral collaboration

Many health issues require the involvement of different government departments or 'sectors'. Government departments and non-governmental organisations dealing with housing, social welfare, education, agriculture, employment, industry, rural development, communications, women's affairs, youth, transport can all affect health in their different ways. Intersectoral collaboration is an essential element of the concept of primary health care and health promotion described in early chapters of this book. You will almost certainly find yourself in a position where you will need to involve other departments in your programmes or influence their policies so that they support your health promotion activities.

HIV/AIDS provides a good example of the importance of intersectoral collaboration. As part of the global mobilisation to tackle this threat many countries established national AIDS control programmes. However evaluations of the impact of these programmes showed that there was a tendency for HIV/AIDS control to be seen as the responsibility of health services. However, the impact of the HIV/AIDS epidemic goes beyond that of health to embrace all aspects of society – especially in the worst-hit countries of Africa and Asia. At a national level it is damaging fragile economies by reducing the output of factories, mines and agriculture. At the community level it is affecting the capacity of schools and health services to provide the necessary care and farmers to supply food. At the family level it is affecting the abilities of families to feed, clothe and look after their members and it is creating a creating a generation of AIDS orphans dependent on others. One of the biggest challenges has been to raise the profile of HIV/AIDS control as a broader development issue in which all sectors are affected and need to work together for joint action.

Although there is widespread agreement about the need for intersectoral collaboration, it can be very difficult to get everyone to work together. Each agency may have different priorities. Staff may have a narrow view of health as something concerning only hospitals and medicines and may not recognise the role their institution can play. They may be suspicious that you are trying to take some of their budget and 'invade' their 'territory'. The priority of many bureaucracies and administrators is often to protect their own organisation!

Campaigns are one way of uniting different groups for a short intensive action to meet agreed objectives. Sustained collaboration between agencies needs a political commitment from the senior management at district and national levels. Some useful strategies to create the mutual understanding, enthusiasm and commitment to work together are listed below.

• When you are trying to involve someone from another department don't just think what you want that person to do for you. See if you can think of ways in which involvement in your programme might benefit *their* work. Find out what are the special needs, pressures and tasks facing that person and what outcomes of joint action might be perceived as beneficial to them. Are there pressures from their senior management that you need to know about? Much can be achieved informally at a local level through: mutually helping each other; supporting each others' activities; and sharing equipment, skills and transport.

• Hold orientation meetings for persons from different departments at the beginning of your health education programme and provide opportunities for participation, discussion and sharing of thoughts on future activities.

• In any initial training, continuing education or workshop activities you are involved in, encourage a *multidisciplinary* mix of participants. Use participatory training methods that encourage exploration of different perspectives, agreements on respective roles, building of mutual trust and a shared vision for the future and a strategy for joint action.

• Create regular opportunities where the different fieldworkers can meet in an informal setting and exchange information on current activities and problems.

Health and safety at work

Work can be dangerous for your health. Depending on their jobs, workers might be exposed to a variety of hazards that include chemicals, dust, vibration, noise and dangerous machinery. We have only just begun to realise

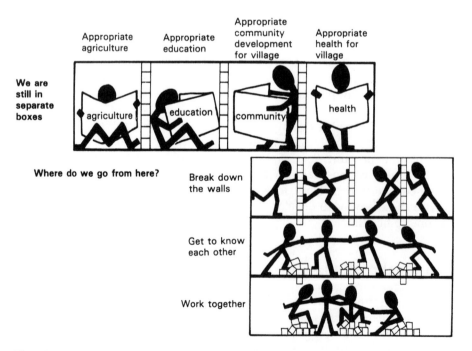

Fig. 10.2 Intersectoral collaboration – breaking the barriers

the harmful effects of many of these. Learning has been a painful process at the expense of many unnecessary deaths.

In 1974 Britain passed its Health and Safety at Work Act that made it law for companies to take action to ensure that their workplace did not have any hazards. Companies had to have a written health and safety at work policy that outlined their strategy and had to appoint a health and safety officer. They were also encouraged to recognise safety representatives nominated by the trade unions and allow them to be released for training. Government officials, called factory inspectors, were given power to enforce this legislation.

This law led to many educational activities. The UK Trades Union Congress set up courses for safety representatives that included the understanding of hazards at the workplace and the nature of the new laws. From the beginning, two opposite perspectives emerged. The management often would blame accidents on 'careless' workers who failed to pay attention, did not wear protective clothing such as goggles or earmuffs, took short cuts in work procedures and broke safety regulations. The workers, on the other hand, took the view that 'work is dangerous for your health'. They blamed accidents on management putting profits before safety by failing to include safety features and using shift work, which affects ability to concentrate. The workers also complained about the lack of information provided about the chemicals and potential toxic hazards that they handled at work. Another example of work practices that can lead to accidents is the use of incentive schemes such as payment per item completed ('piece' work) rather than by the hour. Piece work encourages workers to work faster but also to take more risks, including removal of protective guards, to earn more money.

The British experience raised some important issues. It showed that it was not enough to rely on management's goodwill to ensure that the workplace was safe. Government legislation was needed. However, even with legislation, there were insufficient inspectors to do any more than make the occasional visit to a factory. Enforcement of the law required a strong trade union movement supported by educational activities among management and the workforce.

One of the worst industrial disasters was the explosion in 1984 at the pesticide plant operated by the United States-based Union Carbide Company at Bhopal in India. Deadly methyl isocyanate gas leaked into the atmosphere and killed 2500 persons and injured a further 200,000 people in the surrounding area. In their report on this disaster, the International Confederation of Free Trade Unions (ICFTU) highlighted the fact that the surrounding community was kept ignorant about the potential danger of the chemicals produced. Safety precautions were poor and training in safety inadequate. Most seriously, they found that workers who had earlier complained about safety standards had been punished by transfer to lower paying jobs.

The ICFTU made recommendations which, if implemented could prevent such disasters in future. These included:

- Workers, trade unions and the general public must be given the full facts about the hazards of any chemical plant, the steps taken to prevent accidents and what must be done if an accident does happen.
- The basic rights of workers and their trade unions should be respected within chemical plants. Workers should be able to select their safety representatives through their trade unions. And the workers must have the right, without any fear of reprisal, to refuse any task that they believe might endanger themselves or the public.

One criticism of educational activities at the workplace is that they tend to concentrate on the prevention of accidents and diseases in the workplace. Many now feel that a broader view of health at the workplace is needed. This should include issues such as stress, alcohol consumption, canteen food, smoking policy, crèches for children, and counselling policy. The workplace provides a good opportunity for reaching out to people on a many issues affecting their lives. For example, workplace health education activities in the United Kingdom have included setting up alcohol policies, changing canteen menus, screening pregnant women at work and setting up policies to cover HIV and AIDS.

The issue of health and safety at work in developing countries is only just receiving attention. A particularly difficult problem is the weak state of many trade unions that makes it easy for management to say that they cannot afford safety measures. In a globalised world national governments are often unwilling to enforce safety regulations on foreign-owned factories, which might be moved to another country with fewer restrictions. As long as there is poverty and the threat of unemployment, people will be willing to work long hours in poor facilities, cramped conditions, with dangerous equipment and exposed to hazardous chemicals.

Tobacco and smoking

Three years ago when we started the process of negotiating the Framework Convention on Tobacco Control, I said tobacco addiction is a communicated disease – communicated through advertising, promotion and sponsorship.

Dr Gro Harlem Brundtland,
WHO Director-General

Voluntary codes [by tobacco companies] have proved to be a failure. A World Bank–WHO study, on the other hand, found that interventions like comprehensive advertisement bans and price increases have a measurable and sustained impact on decreased tobacco use.

Joy de Bayer, Tobacco Control Coordinator
at the World Bank

Some appalling statistics were given in Chapter 1 on the tragic rise in tobacco smoking and the resulting future disease burden. Action to prevent smoking is one of the most cost-effective ways of promoting health and a major challenge to us all. Production and sale of cigarettes are controlled by a small group of multinational companies. Now that health education programmes in industrialised countries have been successful in reducing smoking, these companies are expanding sales of cigarettes in

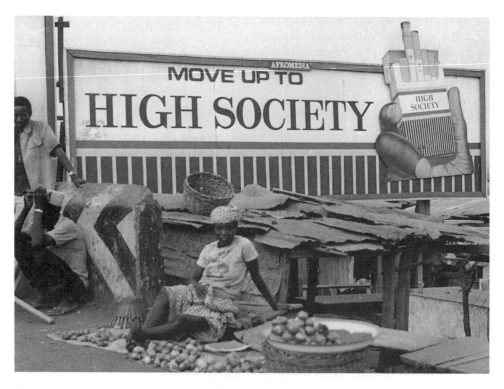

Fig. 10.3 Tobacco advertising in Nigeria

developing countries. They are encouraged by the low levels of health education on smoking, lack of controls on advertising, the increasing incomes of people in the cities and eagerness of governments to have income from tax on tobacco sales. The brands of cigarettes often have much higher levels – often double – of tar and nicotine than the same brands of cigarettes in industrialised nations, where cigarettes with such high levels are banned.

The tobacco companies and their allies are very powerful and influential. Even in industrialised countries it has been difficult to act. Tobacco companies claim that their cigarette advertising is not aimed at encouraging people to smoke, only to switch to their particular brand. However, a careful look at cigarette advertisements shows that this is untrue. Often the advertisements associate cigarettes with modern life, sports, outdoor activities and having fun. In Europe, where advertising of cigarettes has been banned by the government, tobacco companies have switched to sponsorship of events – especially sports. The name of the event has the name of the cigarette brand, which is also displayed prominently on bill-

boards. So every time pictures are shown, or the name of the competition is announced, publicity is given to the tobacco company. When an Indian associate company of the British American Tobacco group sponsored the Indian World Cup Cricket in 1996, a survey showed that smoking among Indian teenagers increased five times. That survey also found that there was an increase among the teenagers of the belief that smoking was good for athletic excellence.

Health educators have been active on smoking for a long time but with only a small part of the money that is available to the tobacco industry. Health education directed at the community is now being supported by the introduction of services such as anti-smoking clinics to help people give up the habit. Most importantly, there has been a shift towards advocacy to encourage countries to pass health-promoting policies that reduce tobacco consumption especially those listed below.

There have been some important success stories in the fight against tobacco companies. The organisation Action on Smoking and Health (ASH) provides an example of the work of a *pressure group* involved in public education and

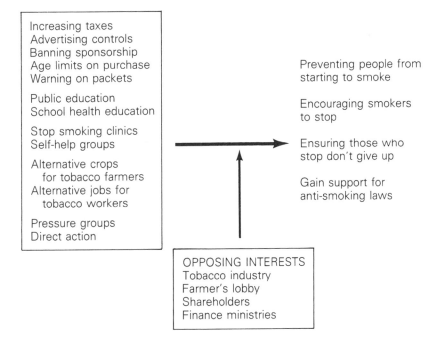

Fig.10.4 Tackling the smoking epidemic

Key actions that WHO suggests governments could undertake to create comprehensive national tobacco control programmes:

- Legislate.
- Ban all tobacco advertising and promotion.
- Ban sales to children.
- Require effective health warnings on all tobacco products.
- Require detailed reporting of constituents of tobacco and tobacco smoke.
- Regulate tobacco products.
- Protect people from involuntary exposure to tobacco smoke by establishing smoke-free public places and workplaces.
- Bring tobacco smuggling under control through stricter law enforcement and improved international cooperation.
- Increase the price of all tobacco products beyond inflation; use part of the revenue for tobacco control, and part to promote economic alternatives to tobacco growing and manufacturing.
- Educate.
- Invest in health education and promotion.
- Provide tobacco-use cessation programmes.
- Support media involvement in the need for tobacco control, the availability of policies that work and the role of the tobacco industry in thwarting implementation of effective tobacco-control policies.
- Counter tobacco industry misinformation campaigns by telling the truth about tobacco.
- Ensure adequate institutional support for tobacco control capacity-building, applied research, routine surveillance and programme evaluation.

itself was a joke as 'bugger up' is a colloquial term for ruining or spoiling. They used humour to challenge the images of health, fitness and sophistication on the advertisements. The public found their slogans funny and newspapers and television gave them publicity and support. The tobacco companies were reluctant to take out legal proceedings against the action group. Newspaper and television reporting of the proceedings of a trial would only provide further publicity to the health hazards of smoking.

As a result of such actions, governments in developed countries have passed laws to ban advertising of tobacco and introduce health warnings on cigarette packages. However, governments in developing countries can be reluctant to pass laws banning tobacco because it will affect their income. For example, almost half the tax collected in Malaysia comes from cigarette sales. In Malawi at least half of the export earnings come from tobacco. Many vested interests have to be overcome to deal with the smoking epidemic! However when governments have the courage to take action, the benefits can be considerable. Thailand introduced comprehensive tobacco control policies in 1992. Smoking prevalence among young Thai adults aged 15–19 dropped from 12.1% to 9.5%, a decline of over one-fifth. Thailand also registered substantial decreases in adult smoking prevalence from 1991 to 1996.

One area of effective action in USA has been to take legal action to sue tobacco companies for the health damages inflicted by smoking. This has been successfully copied in other developed countries. However, successful legal actions in developed countries have strengthened the resolve of tobacco companies to promote their products in developing countries.

One of the most exciting developments in recent years has been the coordinated action by international agencies and the World Health Assembly under the leadership of WHO to establish a Framework Convention on Tobacco Control. The first step to getting this treaty established was in 1996 when the World Health Assembly called upon the Director General of WHO to take steps to promote the concept of a framework convention. This is a legal instru-

influencing media coverage and policy makers. Others have despaired of the reluctance of governments to act on tobacco control and have taken *direct action* that is outside the law. For example, in Australia a group of health educators started writing slogans on the billboards displaying tobacco advertisements. They called themselves Billboard Utilising Graffitists Against Unhealthy Promotion or *BUGA UP*. The name ment with the force of a treaty which will bind signatories to address a wide range of issues including control of tobacco advertising and promotion, agricultural diversification away from growing tobacco, removal of subsidies for tobacco production, and control of smuggling of cigarettes. A draft framework was developed and agreed by the World Health Assembly in 2000. Intensive negotiations with governments then took place and behind the scenes there was considerable pressure both from the international campaigning groups such as ASH and the tobacco industry. An agreed framework convention document was signed at the World Health Assembly in May 2003.

The promotion of bottle-feeding by the infant food industry

In the late 1960s a disturbing trend in many developing countries was observed. Many mothers were turning to bottle-feeding with disastrous consequences for the health of their babies. Lack of water and hygienic facilities for sterilising bottles and teats as well as over-dilution of the baby milk powders led to babies dying from diarrhoea and malnutrition. *A bottle-fed baby in a developing country is 14 times more likely to die in its first year of life than a breast-fed one.*

This trend to bottle-feeding was taking place for several reasons. Working mothers found it difficult to combine breastfeeding with a full-time job. Hospitals and maternity wards often found bottle-feeding more convenient for their routines. A widespread belief was that poor mothers had insufficient milk (although, in reality, fewer than one in a hundred mothers has a medical problem that prevents them from breastfeeding their babies). Many also believed that bottle-feeding was modern and better for their babies. These beliefs had arisen for several reasons. In films and magazines bottle-feeding often appeared and breasts were shown as objects of sex. Mothers wishing to breastfeed were discouraged by maternity hospital procedures such as separation of mother from baby, free samples of baby milk and lack of support by trained staff for women experiencing feeding difficulties.

But the most important reason for the rise in bottle-feeding came from the promotional activities of multinational baby food companies such as Nestlé, Glaxo and Meiji. Their radio, television and billboard advertisements as well as brightly decorated cans of milk promoted the image of bottle-feeding as safe and modern, and undermined women's confidence in breastfeeding. Besides advertising, baby milk companies carried out other promotional activities including giving free samples of baby milk and advertising in hospitals. Some companies even used sales promotion persons dressed in white coats like health workers.

In the 1970s health workers throughout the developing world began to express concern at the way the infant food manufacturers were promoting bottle-feeding. Charities, consumer groups and development agencies such including UNICEF and WHO took up the case. Health workers and women's groups such as the National Childbirth Trust in the United Kingdom were beginning to campaign for a return to breastfeeding in developed countries. So there was the formation of a link and common understanding between countries. An extended international campaign was set up to try to control the activities of the infant food manufacturers. Actions taken included lobbying politicians, law suits, and boycotts of products from companies such as Nestlé.

An important result of the campaigning was the adoption in 1980 by an international gathering of WHO, UNICEF, governments and NGOs of an *International Code for the Marketing of Breast Milk Substitutes* whose provisions included:

- *no free samples or supplies* to be given to mothers or maternity hospitals;
- *no promotion in hospitals* – company posters and literature advertising infant milk products are not allowed in health care facilities;
- *no unscientific promotion to health workers* (including personal gifts) – product literature should be scientific and factual, not promotional;
- *no direct consumer promotion* of infant milk through the mass media and direct contact with customers is prohibited;

- *non-promotional labels* – labels should be non-promotional and include a clear statement on the superiority of breastfeeding and warnings about the hazards of bottle-feeding;
- *scope* – the Code covers breast-milk substitutes, feeding bottles and teats and other products that interfere with breastfeeding.

Individual health workers, development agencies, churches and governments throughout the developing world have mobilised to monitor the implementation of the code. Local self-help groups such as the Baby Milk Action Coalition in United Kingdom, Breast Feeding Information group in Kenya and the BUNSO group in Philippines were formed. They monitor the activities of infant-food manufacturers, promote breastfeeding among the public, train health workers in breastfeeding counselling and campaign to change maternity hospital practices to encourage breastfeeding. The La Lèche League is a network of women who have groups throughout the world promoting breastfeeding. The International Baby Food Action Network (IBFAN) acts as an international resource agency.

The BUNSO group in the Philippines is a good example of a local organisation that is standing up to the baby foods industry (the initials BUNSO are an abbreviation for 'Partnership and Coalition to Save the Infant' in the local language). It is a national coalition of concerned mothers, health workers, consumers, trade union members in the food and drug industry, and church groups. They are engaged in the promotion and protection of breastfeeding and in the defence of women and children's rights to proper health and nutrition. BUNSO acts as a 'watchdog' to the milk industry's marketing practices and monitors practices of hospitals, doctors and health workers. BUNSO was one of the breastfeeding actions groups that, as part of IBFAN, participated in the drafting of the Infant Formula Marketing Code.

On the 20th anniversary of the code, IBFAN produced a report *Breaking the code 2001*, which documented the problems, successes and achievements since the code was launched.

IBFAN reported proof of violations by all of the major baby food companies.

While most companies (but not all!) have removed pictures of baby's faces from tins of milk, a common practice has been to replace them with pictures of cuddly animals or cartoon characters for example Mead Johnson has used the story-book character Peter Rabbit and Nestlé have used a blue bear. Free supplies continue to be given either as gifts to hospitals and through other channels described below. A recent practice by infant food companies has been to set up 'baby clubs' that contact mothers to send promotional materials, free gifts and samples of infant formula. Mothers' wards and waiting rooms continue to display products that contain the marketing logos of baby food companies, such as posters, calendars, clocks and growth charts.

The Internet is a new development and not covered in the Code. Because a web site can be viewed anywhere in the world it is difficult to regulate its content. Examples of Code violations found by IBFAN on Internet web sites included comparisons between their company's products and breast milk (Abbott Ros, Meiji and Mornaga), pictures of babies (Nestlé and Gerber) and offers of free samples, gifts and discounts as incentives to buy infant formula (Gerber, Nestlé Carnation and Mead Johnson).

Among the successes reported by IBFAN was the fact that 51 countries had passed laws that incorporated the provisions of the Code. Some countries even went further than the Code in controlling promotion of infant formula. Brazil, for example, introduced a law that required companies to remove pictures of babies, bottles or animal toys from formula and baby-food labels; and to put clear warnings that the product is not to be used for babies younger than 6 months. In Ghana, laws have been introduced which prohibit the marketing of any product directed at feeding infants up to 6 months of age.

Continued vigilance is needed to monitor the enforcement of the Code and close the loopholes that the infant formula companies are quick to identify and exploit.

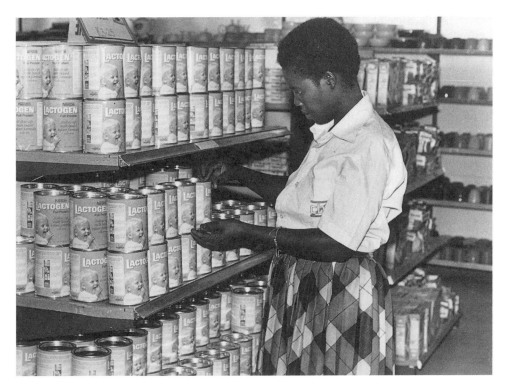

Fig.10.5   Smiling baby on tins of baby milk in Zambia in 1983 – now banned under the International Code for Marketing of Breast Milk Substitutes

The promotion of non-essential drugs by multinational companies

A large proportion of national health budgets goes on purchase of drugs. Today over one-third of the world's population still lacks access to essential drugs in the poorest parts of Africa. Fewer than one in three developing countries have fully functioning drug regulatory authorities. Some 10 to 20% of sampled drugs fail quality control tests in many developing countries. Failure in good manufacturing practices too often results in toxic, sometimes lethal, products. There is increasing concern about the use of drugs that are harmful, unnecessary or which could be available at a much cheaper price if bought as 'generic' drugs rather than branded products offered by the multinational pharmaceutical companies.

In response to this problem WHO launched an Essential Drugs Programme. This is helping countries reduce the cost of importing drugs by concentrating on the supply and use of some 300 drugs considered the most essential. Regularly updated information on the Essential Drugs Programme can be found in the free newsletter *Essential Drugs Monitor* listed in the Appendix.

However, the Essential Drugs Programme has been opposed by the pharmaceutical companies who invest large sums of money in promotion of their drugs through free samples, gifts and incentives to health workers.

One group of drugs that are unnecessary are 'anti-diarrhoeal' medicines. These operate by reducing mobility of the gut. They may relieve symptoms but do not deal with the root causes of diarrhoea. They also distract attention from the life-saving intervention of oral rehydration. Given to young children they can be extremely dangerous. In Pakistan, for example, the company Janssen supplied Immodium (loperamide) in droplet form despite the unsuitability of the drug for infants. Despite protests from doctors about babies dying because of this drug the company only finally stopped the availability of the drug after a British television programme exposed the problem in June 1990.

Health Action International is an informal network of consumer, health, development action and other public interest groups involved in health and pharmaceutical issues in 60 countries around the world. It believes that all drugs marketed should: meet real medical needs, have therapeutic advantages, be acceptably safe and offer value for money.

Besides tobacco, baby milks and diarrhoeal medicines, other commercial products can be dangerous to health including: drugs with harmful side effects, faulty electrical equipment, clothes made from inflammable materials, harmful chemicals in cosmetics such as skin-lightening creams and eye colouring. Consumers International provides a coordinating function for consumer groups throughout the world who are campaigning for safe products (see Appendix).

Advocacy and agenda setting

A priority for advocacy is to get issues on the 'agenda' of politicians so that they will take them seriously and initiate action. The approach to planning we often see in textbooks is one where priorities are decided according to needs. For example, we might look at prevalence of the disease, trends, seriousness and effect on mortality and morbidity. We might also consider the cost of treatment, feasibility of prevention and felt needs of the community. However, decisions by politicians and government officials are rarely made according to this 'rational' planning model. They are usually made in response to different pressures according to: the *status quo* – what has been the practice up to now; influence of friends; allocation of funds from the central government; influence of pressure groups such as professional bodies, commercial companies, trade unions and political parties; external pressures such as prices of imported goods; wishes of aid donor organisations such as the World Bank and the International Monetary Fund; newspapers and television; and public opinion.

Priorities are usually based on short-term pressures and rarely consider longer-term issues such as health and environment. Of course we cannot expect health to be the only issue that governments consider. But we can try to influence the public to support health promotion and ensure that politicians are fully informed about the health implications of their decisions.

Forms of protest and action

Those campaigns described above used many different approaches to influence politicians and multinational companies. I have listed on page 199 many different forms of direct action, protest and campaigning approaches (this list is adapted from a longer list of methods of non-violent action prepared by the American peace activist Gene Sharp). They have been used in campaigns on a wide range of issues including health. Which ones do you think you could apply to bringing attention to a health issue in your community?

The impact of the different methods listed on page 199 depends a great deal on the nature of the health issue and the extent to which the action captures the imagination of the politicians, the media and the public. You can refer to Chapter 8 that describes the type of activities or 'media events' that catch the interest of newspapers, radio and television and explains how to write a press release. People's imagination will be drawn by striking and symbolic acts and the honesty, conviction and sacrifice of those taking action.

One person famous for use of non-violent protests was the Indian Mahatma Gandhi. The methods he used to fight injustice and advance the cause of freedom for India are well worth studying as models of action. He called his approach *satyagraha* which means 'truth force'. He used a range of methods including hunger strikes, boycotts, sit-ins, strikes, mass 'stay at homes' and *civil disobedience* – which is the deliberate breaking of laws and being willing to go to prison for causes that one's conscience feels to be just.

Forms of protest and persuasion

Formal statements
public speeches
letter of opposition/of support
declaration from an organisation
signed public statement
declaration of intention
group or mass petition

**Communication with a
wider audience**
slogans, symbols
banners, posters and displays
leaflets, pamphlets and books
newspapers and journals
records, television and radio

Group representation
sending a deputation
presenting a mock award
group lobbying
picketing

Symbolic public acts
display or wearing of symbols
prayer and worship
delivering symbolic objects
destruction of one's own property
symbolic lights, e.g. candles
display of portraits

Pressure on individuals
frequent visits
letter writing
personal approaches
vigils

Drama and music
humorous sketches,
jokes
performance of plays and music
singing

Processions
marches and parades
religious processions
pilgrimages
honouring the dead
mock funerals
demonstrating at funerals
homage at burial places

Public assemblies
assemblies of protest and support
protest meetings
teach-ins

Withdrawal and renouncing
walkouts
silence
renouncing honours
turning one's back

Boycotts
boycotting of meetings
withdrawing membership from
    institutions
stay at home
total personal non-cooperation
consumer boycott

Strikes
protest strike
industry strike
selective strike
general strike

Civil disobedience
slow compliance
sit-down
civil disobedience

Other non-violent interventions
fasting
sit-ins
stay-in strike
overloading of administration

Globalisation, networking and the power of the Internet

Improvement in health will often depend on individual countries adopting health-promoting policies. However, many of the policies will be affected by events outside the countries – actions by individuals, groups, organisations and nations. Globalisation is the name given to the process by which international forces have come to play an increasing role in shaping our lives.

Globalisation can damage health. In this chapter you have seen some examples of the influence of tobacco, drug and baby-milk com-

panies; the heavy dependence on cash crops; unequal trading conditions; wars and migration; communication and transmission of infections diseases such as AIDS. The harm caused by globalisation has been highlighted by protests and demonstrations at international meetings.

However, globalisation can also open up new possibilities for promoting health. With suitable safeguards, international business can provide resources for investment, international trade agreements such as OPEC for oil can secure fair returns for products. Examples such as the International Code for Marketing of Infant Milk Formulas and the Framework

Convention on Tobacco Control show the potential for international agreements. WHO and the World Health Assembly provide the mechanism by which the countries of the world support each other and coordinate action. Until recently WHO has tended to restrict its work to technical support for country programmes. The Framework Convention on Tobacco Control is WHO's first exercise in international treaty making – and represents a welcome shift in WHO's approach towards a more active advocacy role for global health.

Another positive dimension of globalisation has been the linking together and networking of pressure groups within countries to form global movements for health advocacy, e.g. Health Action International and International Baby Food Action Network. The Internet has become a powerful tool for supporting this networking through the ability to post detailed information and reports on health topics in Internet web sites that can be accessed by everyone, the enhanced opportunities to share information between organisations and as cheap form of communication through e-mail. For most health topics you can find discussion groups with members from throughout the world who share news and information on a daily basis through e-mail. At little expense, it is now possible to have instantaneous contact with thousands of other persons throughout the world to ask for help, 'blow the whistle' on dangerous local practices and agree on coordinated strategies. The Internet has opened up a new era for advocacy for health.

Summary

The promotion of health often involves activities that are 'political' and involve policies of governments. Most programmes to improve health will require some advocacy directed at influencing government policy. Some changes can be achieved in the short-term such as changes in the way existing laws are enforced and policies are implemented. Other changes may only be possible in the long term such as introduction of new laws and removal of outdated laws. Advocacy directed at influencing policy is an essential strategy in the armoury of health promotion. This chapter has described how people and groups have tried to make governments and multinational companies adopt health promoting policies. Some of the lessons are:

- There may be little you can do on your own. Find people with more influence and power who will support your case.
- Try and persuade respected bodies such as professional associations and churches to pass resolutions and take up the case.
- It's always easier to ignore, discipline and attack individuals. If you are dealing with something controversial it is better to have your views coming from a *group* of people rather than named individuals who can be exposed and publicly criticised.
- It's much easier for officials to ignore criticism if no evidence is presented. So always support your case with accurate information. Include specific examples, with testimonies and photographs, of the harm that is being done by a particular policy.
- Newspapers and other media can be used to promote your case and you should be prepared to brief journalists, stage 'media events' and prepare press releases.
- Issues often have international dimensions and involve multinational companies. In this case you should form links with groups in other countries and international agencies. You should harness the power of the e-mail and the Internet to link up with others who feel the same way you do and who will support you. Some useful addresses are provided in the Appendix of this book.
- If your cause is a just one, you will have the support of a network of well-wishers within your country and abroad. Don't give up!

<table>
<tr><td>

11

</td><td>

Putting it into practice

</td></tr>
</table>

By now, if you have followed the earlier chapters in this book, you should be able to determine the contribution of health education, service improvement and advocacy to human behaviour and health, and choose methods and strategies for achieving these changes. This chapter will describe how you can put everything together into a planned programme of activities and:

1   set objectives;
2   look at needs, researching the problem, developing a strategy;
3   monitor and evaluate your work;
4   make a workplan and prepare a plan/project proposal;
5   implement and manage the programme.

The planning process

Imagine that you are about to take a journey. You know where you are and have to decide where it is you want to go. Then you must decide the best way of getting to your destination. If you do not arrive at the place you wanted to go you realise that you are lost.

Planning a health education programme is like planning a journey. Your starting point is the present health situation, e.g. level of immunisation, sanitation. Your destination is the level of improvement you would like to reach. To do this you must decide on a *strategy* – the methods you must use to improve the situation. At the end you evaluate your programme to find out if you have reached your target – or have got lost!

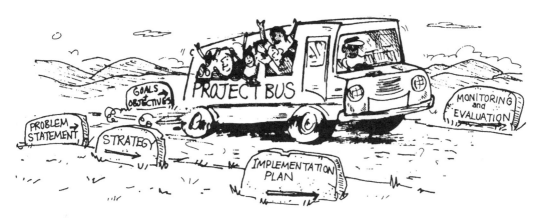

Fig.11.1   Planning a programme is like planning a journey

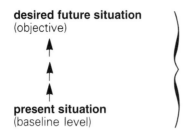

Fig. 11.2   The planning process

When you plan your programme, you are making four sets of decisions:

- Decisions on the present situation – *where are we now?*
- Deciding desired future outcome – *where do we want to go?*
- Decisions on methods or strategy – *how will we get there?*
- Decisions on evaluation strategy – *how will we know when we get there?*

A good way of finding out the present situation is to carry out a community profile or 'diagnosis' as described in Chapter 6. Setting objectives involves making decisions about how much improvement of the present situation is needed and what can be achieved within the time, money and resources available.

In earlier chapters, I showed that we can predict the likelihood of promoting a particular action through an understanding of the economic and cultural influences as well as the felt needs of the community. The amount of change you can expect to achieve will depend on the: *nature of your proposed changes* (Are they simple to perform? Do they fit in with existing practices? Do they fit in with the felt needs of the community?); and *your available resources* (time, personnel and money).

You should *consider alternative methods* and their likely effectiveness before choosing the one that is most suited to your situation. In Chapter 3, guidelines were given on the likely effectiveness of different methods. A useful guide to deciding how much you can achieve is to find out how much change took place in similar settings with other programmes.

How free are you to try out new ideas? Are there any restrictions on your actions from your job description, situation, pressure from employers and the policies of your government? One important restraint is the extent to which you are able to work with fieldworkers from other departments and non-governmental organisations. As described in Chapter 10, intersectoral collaboration is necessary to tackle economic and social issues, such as housing, education, agriculture, community development, employment and women's rights.

In setting targets for change you should be ambitious and try to achieve as much as possible – but also realistic!

Aims and objectives

Aims are general statements of what the programme is trying to achieve such as:

To eliminate child poverty.
To improve the health of children in Chikoko District.
To increase the number of people using latrines.

Aims are statements of intent and not expressed in a measurable way. Many wonder why bother to include them in documents at all! As general statements they can be useful in getting everyone to agree about a common purpose. However, more specific statements are needed when planning programmes. An 'objective' – also called a 'target' – is a statement of proposed change over a fixed time period. An objective should be *measurable*. Setting measurable objectives will enable you to:

- let others know exactly what you are planning;
- make decisions about implementation; and
- evaluate the programme.

Another word for objective is a target. There can be much confusion in the way people use these terms. Some people use the word goal instead of aim, others use objective to describe a general statement of intention! However, it doesn't really matter what terms you use providing that you can recognise the difference between a general and a detailed measurable statement of planned activities. Make sure that you always include specific statements of proposed changes in *your* plan.

Intermediate and impact objectives

You can set objectives for the intended *outcomes* of the programme. It is also useful to set objectives for the completion of activities required to achieve your desired outcome. These are sometimes called operational – or process – objectives. Later in this chapter you will see how these operational objectives can be displayed on a workplan and bar chart and used to monitor a programme.

outcome objectives:	improvements in health
	changes in behaviour
	changes in knowledge, beliefs, attitudes
	empowerment
operational objectives:	initial surveys
	formation of organising committee
	training of key workers
	field visits
	broadcasting of radio programmes
	testing of educational materials
	printing of publications
	purchase of equipment
	completion of health education activities
	evaluation surveys

Writing measurable objectives

An objective (also called a target) for a communication should specify:

- the **intended change** in a detailed measurable form, e.g. acquire facts, develop decision-making ability, change beliefs, change behaviour, learn a practical skill, completion of the training programme;
- the **amount of change** above the initial baseline level, e.g. the percentage able to demonstrate to the interviewer the correct method for making oral rehydration solution should increase from 10 to 50%;
- **who** the communication should be directed at (including where they live) – often called the 'target audience', e.g. grandmothers in Eastern Province, adult men in Lusaka, church ministers in whole country, teachers in Chingleput District, women with one child in Yunan Province;
- the **time scale** over which the desired change should take place, e.g. over the next 12 months;
- changes that are **relevant** and **realistic**.

One way of remembering the characteristics of good objectives is to use the word SMART: **S**pecific, **M**easurable, **A**chievable, **R**elevant, **T**ime bound.

Some problems with objectives

If objectives are so important, why are some people afraid to set them? This can be for several reasons. The present situation may be so uncertain that there is no data for which to set an initial baseline or make sensible decisions on what can be achieved. Then, the best strategy would be to plan some research and data gathering at the start. Once data are available you can set objectives for the remaining period of the plan.

Some people feel that, if you honestly believe in community participation, it is wrong to set objectives as these should come from the community. However, in Chapter 6 you were shown how to set objectives for *processes* within a community participation approach, such as the formation of committees and reaching group decisions.

One reason for not setting objectives is that people may feel threatened by openly stating their objectives. They may feel that others will criticise them if they fail to reach the targets. It is important therefore to set objectives that are realistic for the problem you are trying to solve and the resources at your disposal. Even so, failing to reach objectives is not something to be ashamed of – provided you evaluate and find out why the activities failed and avoid those mistakes in future activities.

Research in health education and health promotion

One important reason many health education programmes fail is that the activities undertaken were planned with a poor understanding of the problem. Research involves the *systematic* collection of information (often called 'data') *to answer particular questions*. In earlier chapters you saw how important it was to understand your community and its special needs. Selection of what factors to change, choice of communication methods and content of messages should be determined from characteristics of the intended audience. Some of the areas where research can help you to plan your health education and health promotion activities are shown in Table 11.1.

Community profile

You may only need information on part of your community, e.g. out-of-school youths or the whole community. The term community profile, or 'community diagnosis', was introduced in Chapter 6 and is the process by which you systematically obtain information to understand the community in which you plan to work.

A community profile may be needed for many reasons. It can help you decide where to put your health education effort by letting you know special needs, e.g. children, elderly, families with young children, the disabled and poor. A profile might be needed to provide evidence to convince others of the need for a special programme. However the usual reason for making

Table 11.1 The role of research in communication programmes

Problem definition	Community surveys to determine the level of disease/trends and felt needs of the community
Determining role of human behaviour	Surveys of community practices; research on prevention and control of disease
Understanding influences on community behaviour	Surveys to determine influences on behaviour; sources of knowledge; role and origins of beliefs; influential persons in family and community; economic and social barriers to action
Decisions on communication	Surveys to determine communication systems in community
Strategy	Familiarity and exposure to different media; characteristics of target groups; effectiveness of different media; opinion leaders that can be used in the programme
Programme implementation	Pre-testing of messages and materials; evaluation of training; development of education methods; monitoring of progress
Evaluation and feedback	Evaluation research

a community profile is to plan a community-based health education programme.

The research process

Research is often seen as a complicated process that needs a lot of time, detailed understanding of statistics and access to facilities such as computers. As a result many people feel that they cannot do research and just base their activities on what they

FLOW CHART FOR AN EPIDEMIOLOGICAL INVESTIGATION

Lovel, H.J. (1980) Institute of Child Health, London WClN 1EH

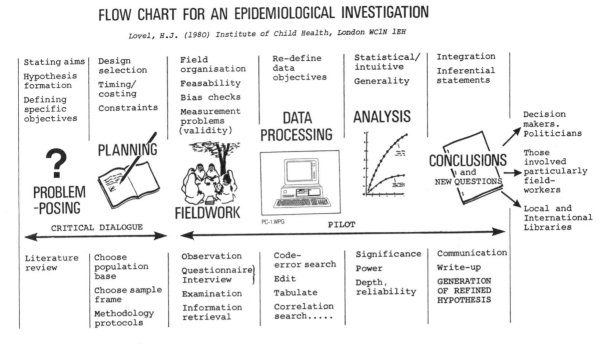

Fig. 11.3   The research process

---

feel is the right approach. But, as you saw in earlier chapters, our training and background may set us apart from the community. It can be difficult for to imagine how a young child, old person, poor villager or member of the opposite sex really feels. We can easily be mistaken if we only rely on our own judgement and do not try to find out what people really feel about these topics.

You can still obtain worthwhile information using simple research methods that do not need large amounts of time and money. You can find out more about research methods in Marie Therese Feuerstein's excellent handbook *Partners in Evaluation* (see Appendix).

Deciding what information to find out

Planning a piece of research involves making decisions about:

- what information is required;
- how that information should be collected to obtain a true picture of the situation and to avoid bias and errors.

A starting-point for any research is to make a list of the questions that you want to answer.

In making that list you can draw from many sources. Your experience or that of other field-workers may suggest topics to explore. Reports of the findings of other programmes might suggest issues to consider. Behavioural science concepts or particular theories may also suggest certain kinds of information needed – for example the checklist of questions about social influence and health beliefs on pages 31 and 34. Some questions will be determined by your topic, e.g. you may have to find out how many elderly people there are in a community and where they live. The types of information to answer these questions are listed on page 206.

Deciding how to obtain the information

The data collection methods you use should provide the information you need and give a real picture of the situation. Some of the mistakes to avoid are: only believing data when it fits in with what you think is going on; people telling you what they want you to know, and not the actual truth – they may deliberately hide the truth or just find your questions confusing and difficult to answer; and asking

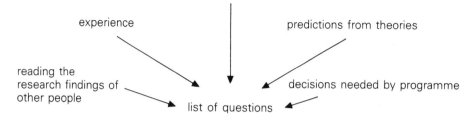

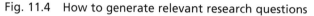

Fig. 11.4 How to generate relevant research questions

Types of information required in communication research

Basic information on the community, such as size and composition of the population, at-risk groups, income, educational level, religion, social class.

Needs of the area. Needs may be those identified by the health educator using medical criteria. They may be expressed needs that have already been put forward by the community or by the voluntary and government workers in the area or felt needs that have not yet been expressed. Many projects fail because they do not pay enough attention to expressed and felt needs of the communities.

Existing channels of communication within a community. These may be informal channels such as neighbourhood social networks, opinion leaders, shopkeepers, tea shop; or formal channels such as schools, health workers, community workers, youth leaders. Also important are details of what media are available and popular, e.g. newspapers, magazines, radio and television programmes. Find out what health information is already being conveyed through these existing channels of communication. Does it agree or contradict your own messages? Can you mobilise these communication channels?

Influences on health behaviour. These were described in Chapter 2. Influences may operate at the individual, family, community level or higher level. They include: the physical conditions of the area such as housing, environment and the availability and quality of services such as clinics and schools; the local norms, attitudes, values and knowledge that make up the community culture; and the power structure both formal through elected politicians and officials, and informal, through community leaders, opinion leaders and significant others.

Baseline data for evaluation. Information gathered at the initial stage of making the community profile provides the baseline data to set objectives and evaluate your programme.

Guidelines for avoiding bias in research

- Use more than one method or source of information and then check if the information obtained from the different methods agree – this is called 'triangulation'.
- Choose the people you talk to (your 'sample') to make sure that they are *representative,* e.g. for age, sex, education, income, of the group you are investigating. Do not just interview people who are easier to contact, e.g. who live nearby, or come to clinics. One way of sampling the population is to make a *random* sample. For example you could write down the names of all the people on separate sheets of paper and pick them out of a box. Another simple approach is to select every third house you come across (although in some cases that might result in biases).
- Take time to explain why you are finding out the information. People are more likely to answer you truthfully if they trust you and believe that you are going to use the information to help them. Be honest about how you will use the information and emphasise that any information provided will be confidential. It may be better to ask someone else to do the interviewing if you think that it will provide more truthful answers: for example you can use

a young person to interview another young person, a woman to interview a woman; an older person to interview an older person.

- Find out whether in your community there are subjects that are considered taboo and impolite to talk about and ask questions. If this is the type of information you are trying to find out, you will have to consider carefully how you can ask these questions. One approach is to emphasise the confidentiality of the information.

- Avoid leading persons to answer in particular ways by the questions you ask. Explain that you really are interested in what they *themselves* think. Wherever possible, ask open questions that allow people to give frank opinions in their own words and tell you what *they* think is important.

- Involve the local communities themselves in planning the survey and doing the interviewing. This approach is called *participatory research*. This is a good way to encourage community participation and ensure that the community profile includes data that the local community see as important (see Chapter 6 on Working with communities).

the views of a small group of people who do not represent the whole community. You can avoid many of these problems by following the guidelines listed here.

Qualitative and quantitative research

Quantitative research methods collect specific information and facts that can be expressed as numbers. The numbers can then be treated mathematically to produce overall data for the community, e.g. number of households with latrines, number of children, specific knowledge about nutrition, numbers of people who hold a particular belief about the spread of AIDS. Quantitative information can be obtained through observation by looking for specific practices. Quantitative data can also be obtained from questionnaires and interviews that ask 'closed' questions. These are questions which have to be answered in a specific way, with numbers, by saying yes or no or agreeing/disagreeing with statements on a list.

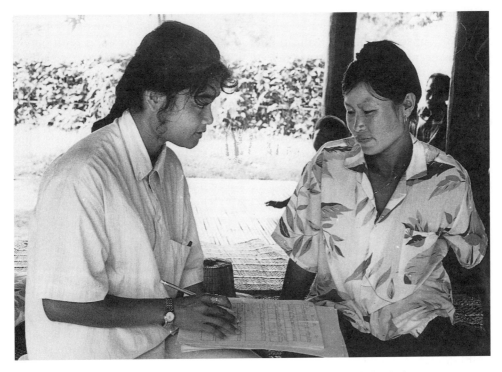

Fig. 11.5   Careful choice of questions is needed to avoid bias and obtain honest answers

open-ended question	*What do you think are the causes of diarrhoea?*
closed question	*Do you agree that diarrhoea is caused by teething?* *Yes/no*

Qualitative research methods ask 'open-ended' questions where the community answer in their own words and are given freedom to expand and give their thoughts on the subject. Interviews and observation are used as well as focus group discussions. Qualitative research methods can give rich insights into the local situation and people's feelings. But it is difficult to summarise the information obtained and get a complete picture of a community. Interpretation of qualitative data depends a great deal on the honesty and skill of the person doing the interviews. It is easy to introduce bias by letting your own feelings and interests influence how you interpret the data.

Qualitative research is particularly useful for 'rapid appraisals' of the situation. It is also used a great deal in helping to develop appropriate communication messages. You can find out the views of young people, test out (or 'pre-test') media such as posters, radio programmes and get a feel for the impact of a health education programme. However, quantitative data is necessary if you have to get some idea of the size of a problem or need to convince policy-makers of the need to take action.

In practice it is best to try to include a combination of qualitative and quantitative methods. One approach is to use qualitative approaches to get a 'feel' for the situation and to identify issues for follow-up study in quantitative surveys.

Sources of data

Published sources and records and interviews with field staff

Start with existing sources such as the Census, previous surveys and records and files of agencies operating in the area. It is surprising how much useful information can be obtained from the most unlikely sources such as government reports, minutes of meetings and newspaper reports. However, much of the available information can be of poor quality, irrelevant and out of date. Health data from clinic and hospital data can give a useful picture of the local situation but only represent cases where people have come for treatment. They will miss out cases that people have treated at home or taken to private or traditional healers.

Look out for field staff from health and other services who have worked in the community and can give you the benefit of their experience. Try to speak to some of them and see if they agree with each other and with what the community themselves say.

Interviews in the community

The next stage of data collection is to go to the area and meet the people who live and work there. But be careful – surveys can be expensive and time-consuming and arouse expectations of action that you may not be able to fulfil.

It is often more efficient to interview informally members of the community and workers in various government and voluntary organisations – the 'key informants'. This provides information about the area and is an opportunity to introduce yourself and your health education interests. Give careful thought to the people you can interview to get a balanced and true picture. Your informants might give different and contradictory responses. But even these differences can tell you a great deal, as it is important to understand the conflicts and tensions within the community. Leaving out a key person may also cause problems later if they feel that their views are being ignored!

Focus group discussions

These are discussions with groups of people in the community carried out in a systematic way to provide information on a topic. Groups of people sharing the same characteristics are brought together. A group discussion is guided by questions asked by the interviewer. These should be open-ended and designed to make people respond and discuss. You should try to limit your own involvement to that of a facilitator. You should encourage discussion *between* the group members so you can observe the language used and feelings of the group.

Observation

Another way to get to know a community is 'street work' or observation. This involves casual observations and informal conversations with residents of the area on doorsteps, public places, shops etc. It is also possible to have 'structured' observation with a checklist of points to look out for so that the observation is carried out in a systematic way – see the list here for an example of an observational checklist.

Intervention-based approaches

A good approach is to carry out some health promotion on a small scale and learn from people's reactions. For example you can find out the feelings of the community by carrying out some health education and asking for comments and feedback. You can ask people's opinions

---

Health practices observational checklist developed for *Mtu Ni Afya* radio health education project in Tanzania

1. Is there vegetation growing near the house?
2. Are there depressions, holes, or receptacles of any kind near the house that could hold stagnant water?
3. Is there mosquito netting over the bed(s) in the bedroom(s)?
4. Is there mosquito netting on the windows?
5. Is there a latrine that meets *Mtu Ni Afya* standards?
6. Does the latrine have a cover?
7. Is the latrine being used?
8. Is the courtyard around the house free of rubbish?
9. Are there any animal faeces near the house?
10. Are there any rats, other vermin or other pests visible in or around the house?
11. Does the house have any windows?
12. Are there a lot of flies in or around the house?

---

about a leaflet, poster or show a film. You might try setting up an advice stall and monitor what requests for information come from the community. This approach is often used to test new products, e.g. coloured condoms and insecticide-impregnated mosquito nets.

Participatory research

Chapter 6 introduced the concept of participatory research and showed how participatory rural appraisal (PRA) methods could be used in the initial phases of community participation programmes. Through the direct involvement of communities, participatory research methods can provide accurate information about communities and a way of involving communities in actions to improve their situation.

As shown in Figure 11.6, PRA, together with community self-surveys and participatory research are one end of a continuum of research methods that can be used to assess community health needs. PRA is most suited for small-scale interventions and when resources are available to follow-up the PRA with programmes in the community. If you are planning to work on a large scale and want information on the size of a problem to help choose a policy, then more conventional methods using surveys as described below will be appropriate. Surveys using qualitative data, focus group discussions and rapid assessment methods occupy the mid ground – simpler to carry out than full surveys yet still providing rich insights into communities.

Planning a survey

Surveys can use any of the data collection methods described above on all, or a sample, of the people in a community. Before doing a full-scale survey of a community it's better to carry out first a small-scale 'pilot' with interviews and focus group discussions so you already have an idea of the important topics to include and try out the questions. In planning your survey, you can follow the steps in Figure 11.3 and the list of 'Questions to ask'.

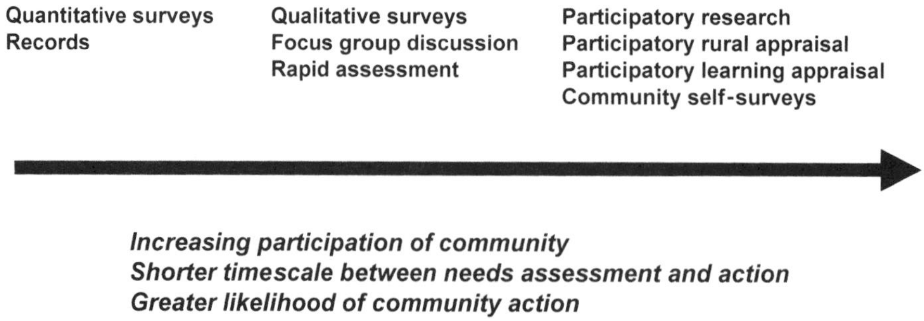

Quantitative surveys	Qualitative surveys	Participatory research
Records	Focus group discussion	Participatory rural appraisal
	Rapid assessment	Participatory learning appraisal
		Community self-surveys

→

Increasing participation of community
Shorter timescale between needs assessment and action
Greater likelihood of community action

Fig. 11.6   Assessing community health needs

Questions to ask in planning community health surveys

Stage 1: Define aims and scope of the study
Why do you need to undertake the survey? What are the needs and problems to be investigated? How will you use the information obtained? Can the information be obtained in any other way?

Stage 2: Decide upon the information requirements
What information is required to deal with the community's needs and problems?
What information is needed for proposing a solution or for allocating resources to the health and community needs?
What do the local fieldworkers feel you should include in the survey?
What do the community feel you should include in the survey?
If funds are limited, what should be the most important questions to ask?

Stage 3: Find out whether the required information is already available
Has a survey already been carried out in the community that might contain useful information? Are there any books or published reports that deal with a similar need in other communities, at a regional or at a national level?

Stage 4: Assess whether the survey can succeed
Will a survey provide the information you need? Are there sufficient resources (money, field staff) and time to carry out the survey?

Stage 5: Making decisions on data collection, sampling and implementation
How will the data be collected – observation, interviews, focus group discussions?
If using observation, what will you include in the checklist? If asking questions what wording will you use and how will you test the questions to make sure they are understood and acceptable?
How are the communities and people in the sample to be selected? How many are to be included? How long will each interview/observation visit take?
When will the data collection take place – time of day, day of week, season? How long will the survey take to complete?
Who will you use to carry out the interviewing? Can you involve local fieldworkers, volunteers or members of the community? Will they need training?
What arrangements are needed to get the interviewers to the field?
How are you going to involve the community in your survey?
How much time is needed to complete all the fieldwork including visiting and interviewing?
How will you analyse and present the data?

Stage 6: Estimating the cost of the survey and preparing a budget
How much will it cost to undertake the survey including transport, staffing and other help?
Are there non-essential questions that can be left out of the survey to reduce the cost? Could the number of people or geographical area of the sample be reduced?

Monitoring and evaluation

Evaluation is the systematic and scientific process determining the extent to which an action or set of actions were successful in the achievement of pre-determined objectives. It involves measurement of adequacy, effectiveness and efficiency of health services.

WHO (1969)

We evaluate to aid future planning and to improve programmes, to increase our understanding of health education practice, to add to the body of knowledge upon which our work is based. We evaluate to achieve operational efficiency and, related to this, to obtain data that permit interpretation of programme effectiveness so as to obtain administrative support, community support and even functional support. We evaluate for reasons associated with motivation – to give staff and volunteers satisfaction, and a sense of success. To give priority to these purposes...we evaluate primarily to study the effects of practice so that we can turn our findings back into practice and improve it and, at the same time, strengthen the scientific basis of practice in health education

Beryl Roberts (1962).

We evaluate communication and health education programmes for many reasons. The most important reason is to learn from our experiences and to improve our methods. The health education methods described in this book have been developed in many different countries and may not work in other situations. You will need to find out what will work in *your own* setting. Health education can only develop as a serious discipline if we build up experience from evaluated programmes.

But there are other important reasons: you may need to evaluate your programmes to show that you are doing your job properly; you may need to justify the money you have received from a funding body; people around you may not believe that health education works and you may need to convince them to give you their support. So evaluations are done for many reasons – some open and others hidden. You will need to decide at the outset *why* you are evaluating your programme and *who* the evaluation is intended for. Some important terms used in evaluation are given below:

- *effectiveness* – whether or not a programme achieves its stated objectives, i.e. did it work?
- *efficiency* – the amount of effort in terms of time, manpower, resources and money required to reach the objectives – was it worth the effort?
- *formative evaluation* – 'monitoring' progress during the programme involving measurement of intermediate objectives, i.e. what have we achieved so far?
- *summative evaluation* – measurement of impact or change at the end of the programme, i.e. have we achieved our objectives?

Evaluation involves showing that:

- *change* has taken place;
- the change took place as a *result* of the programme;
- the amount of *effort* required to produce the change was worthwhile.

So, evaluating your health education involves making some important decisions. What changes to measure? How to measure those changes? How to prove that the changes took place as a result of the programme? Decisions about what changes to measure and how to measure them are really decisions about what should be your *objectives*. These were discussed in an earlier section of this chapter.

Most people would agree that it is important in evaluation to show that change has taken place. But the need to show that change took place as a result of your programme is less obvious. Consider the following situations where external factors had an influence on a programme:

1 An increase in immunisation takes place because a government minister makes a broadcast in the middle of your field campaign.
2 An influential person returns from the city and starts to encourage villagers where you are doing your sanitation programme.
3 In the middle of your AIDS education campaign a famous film star dies of AIDS and this leads to more people adopting safer sex.
4 Diarrhoea rates drop during the 4 months of the programme – but this would have taken

place anyway because of the normal seasonal fall after the rainy season.

Does it really matter that other factors helped your programme? Perhaps not. But what if your programme was an experimental pilot project testing out a new approach that you want to repeat elsewhere? You would have to make certain that the improvements made really had come about because of your new methods and not for other reasons. Otherwise money and effort would be wasted repeating methods that do not actually work!

One reason evaluation is difficult is that it is often only at the end of a programme that thought is given about how the programme should be evaluated. In fact, you should plan at the beginning how you will evaluate your work.

Communication stages and evaluation

It is always best to anticipate problems by 'pretesting' communications with samples of the intended audience before you begin your main activities. However, it is still important to evaluate the programme at the end to find out how effective you have been. In Chapter 3 you saw how communications can fail at many stages – from reaching the sense organs, up to changing health. Communication failure can take place at each of the six stages. If you ask the following questions and find out at which stage a failure in communication took place, you can correct the fault and improve the programme.

Questions to ask when evaluating communication activities

Were the communication activities carried out?
How many radio programmes were broadcast; talks/training sessions given; community meetings held; leaflets distributed; posters put up?

Did the intended audience come across the message?
How many people saw the posters, were able to receive the radio broadcasts, come to the talks, passed by the exhibition?

Did the intended audience pay attention to the communication?
What was the 'coverage' of the programme – how many people saw the poster, listened to the radio programme, stopped to look at the exhibition, were paying attention at the meeting?

Did the intended audience understand the messages?
How many people could correctly repeat back the messages on the posters, radio programmes, talks, meetings?

Did it convince the audience?
How many people accepted and believed the message?

Did it result in change in behaviour?
How many people changed their behaviour as a result of the communication?

Did it lead to improvements in health?
How many people's health improved as a result of the programme?
What changes in level of disease incidence/prevalence took place?

You should be realistic over what changes to look for in your evaluation. Changes in knowledge, understanding, awareness and belief might take place soon after the communication. However, changes in behaviour and health usually take longer to achieve. It is a good idea to carry out a *short-term evaluation* fairly soon after the activity and a *follow-up evaluation* afterwards to look for long-term changes.

Showing that change took place because of your programme

If the objectives have been clearly defined at the outset it is not usually difficult to show that change has taken place your community. However, it is much more difficult to show that it took place *because of your own efforts* and not because of another reason. There are two ways of showing that change was caused by your own efforts (this is called proving 'causality'): see Figure 11.7.

You can set up another group, e.g. another classroom, group of mothers, another village as a 'control' who do not receive the education.

The two groups should be as close as possible in age, education and income. If the group that received your educational programme achieves a better performance than the control group, this will provide strong evidence for the success of your communication activities.

If it is not possible to set up a control group you will have to use an indirect method for excluding other reasons for any changes. You could look carefully at what has taken place – could there be any other possible explanation for the changes that took place? You could interview samples of the community and ask them why they changed their behaviour – was it because of your activities or were there other reasons that you were not aware of?

Process evaluation

This term is used for approaches to evaluation that place more emphasis on the process of the programme and less on achievement of specific outcomes. Typical process activities determined in these kinds of evaluation include the operation of fieldworkers, the collaboration between field agencies, involvement of community organisations and NGOs and overall satisfaction of the community. Many people see process evaluation as a part of the monitoring process (see below). Others see it as distinct from monitoring and

especially appropriate for community-based interventions where objectives are not fixed but evolve during the course of the programme.

Participatory evaluation

Participatory evaluation – described in Chapter 6 – is a form of process evaluation that places special emphasis on involvement of communities. Involvement of the community in evaluation helps to create a bond of trust with the community: you can find out their feelings about the benefits and weaknesses of your activities; you can draw on their experiences and insights on what has happened; evaluation becomes a learning process and the community is able to reflect on its experiences and plan future activities.

Monitoring

Monitoring or 'formative evaluation' takes place during a programme to check that everything is going according to the plan. If problems do occur it is important to find out as soon as possible so you can take action to correct them. Wherever possible, data collection for monitoring (and also evaluation) should be built into routine and on-going activities for management and supervision. Some common sources of data and guidelines for evaluation are given here.

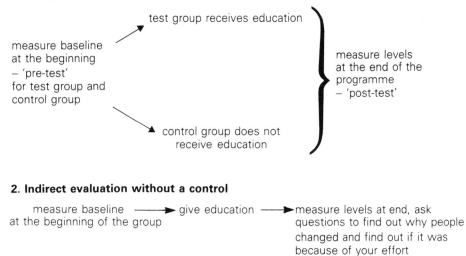

Fig. 11.7   Two approaches to evaluation

Sources of data for monitoring

- **Clinic records/Disease notification** (either as part of case management or surveillance). Useful for measures of service uptake, adherence by patients to advice and effectiveness of treatment. Their value depends on the quality and consistency of record keeping so training and supervisory visits are needed to ensure quality. Data in records are a measure of utilisation of services, and do not always reflect prevalence in the community.
- **Stock records,** e.g. supplies of condoms, drugs, needles. This is a useful measure for measuring uptake of materials (which is not the same as effective use!).
- **Outreach worker contact sheets.** Notes completed by outreach workers/peer educators on activities and educational sessions. These can be a valuable source of data on delivery of intervention, impact and problems experienced. Care is needed to keep forms simple to fill out and to check that they are properly completed.
- **Supervisory visits** carried out as part of an ongoing management of programme to observe performance and discuss their experiences and needs. These can provide useful information on views of field staff, quality of services and what is actually happening. Supervisors can discuss with field staff, observe them in action and record findings on record forms. A supervisor can set up surprise visits, send 'dummy' patients to try out a service, or carry out exit interviews.
- **Focus group discussions** carried out by a trained facilitator with groups of 6–8 persons from the target audience. This is a particularly useful method as it is can be undertaken quickly and cheaply and gathers valuable insights into problems and solutions. It requires a trained facilitator and careful selection of the people to be included in the focus groups.
- **Exit interviews.** Interviews with persons immediately after visiting health services. This can be a useful method for obtaining information on the quality of services and also for evaluating the impact of training and other service improvements.

Summary guidelines for monitoring and evaluation

- Decide at the beginning of a programme how you are going to evaluate it.
- Prepare a set of realistic, achievable and measurable indicators for success. Consult your employers, funding bodies and the community when you decide on your objectives.
- Wherever possible, set up controls groups who do not receive the education. If controls are not possible, collect data that will help you to show that it was your efforts that led to improvements.
- Look for changes in the short term as well as long term. Find out if any benefits are long-lasting.
- Do not limit yourself to just finding out if you have reached your objectives – look out for any unplanned benefits or unexpected problems.
- Look out for ways of involving the target groups in the all stages of the monitoring and evaluation process including setting objectives, collecting data, judging outcomes and deciding on future activities.
- Set up a monitoring system that will keep you informed how the project is working and alert you as soon as any problem occurs so you can take action to deal with it. A good monitoring strategy will also gather much of the data you need for evaluation.
- Learn from your failures as well as successes. Find out why programmes succeeded or failed and what lessons can be drawn for the future.
- Share your successes or failures with others. Tell others about what you have been doing, circulate any reports and look out for newsletters and journals to which you can send articles for publishing.

Managing the programme

This will involve answering the following questions.

- How will you manage your own time and that of the people for whom you are responsible?

- How will you coordinate and support the activities of the different field staff and organisations taking part and involve them in decisions on future activities?
- How will you communicate new information, skills and changes of policy to all involved?
- How will you ensure that the findings from any monitoring and research activities are acted upon as quickly as possible?
- How will you maintain community participation throughout the programme?

Even if your work only involves a few simple activities, it is still worthwhile planning your time. This helps you to use your time efficiently, spreads your workload, anticipates needs and avoids last minute panic. A simple solution to this is to write intended activities on a calendar and circle important days. You can buy or draw for yourself a 'year planner'. This is a large sheet with a square for each day of the year on which you can write key activities using colours to show particular tasks.

Other useful approaches are to set out your objectives as a 'time-line' or a 'bar chart' (sometimes called 'Gantt' chart) for a particular programme on which you can show dates for completing planned activities (see Figure 11.8 and the communication strategy in Figure 3.15). You can also set out a workplan as a table that sets out for each planned activity: the person responsible for carrying out the activity, the date for completion, how you will measure achievement and cost.

A common problem in health education is that fieldworkers give different and conflicting advice, and workers and the community become confused as to what exactly they should do. So you must ensure that everyone is briefed to give the correct information.

At the outset of the programme it is a good idea to run a training workshop to brief those involved, provide any necessary information and give an opportunity to learn any new communication skills.

You will need to maintain the momentum and enthusiasm of your programme. People are more likely to support your programme and put effort into activities if they think that you are taking an interest in what they are doing and are supporting them with advice and resources.

One way to keep in touch is to arrange a regular schedule of visits to different groups. However, the amount of travelling can be reduced if you bring people together for regular meetings to introduce new ideas, review progress and decide future actions. You can carry out your meetings in an effective way by applying the principles of group dynamics that were outlined in Chapter 5.

The discussion on monitoring provided earlier in this chapter suggested some of the ways in which you can collect information about progress achieved by your activities. Supervision visits to fieldworkers in their work settings are especially useful because they provide an opportunity to see how they are getting on, whether lessons from training are being put into practice, to identify problems and provide support. You cannot just assume that because certain tasks are supposed to be carried out that they are really happening!

In addition to meetings with field staff you will need to set up meetings once or twice a year with your employers, senior persons in the various agencies participating in the project and the funding body. This formal management group would review the progress, receive reports and financial statements.

The benefits of community participation were discussed in Chapter 6 and it is important that your management strategy includes setting up opportunities for community involvement. Your field visits should include meetings with communities, who can also be invited to send representatives to your management group meetings.

Plan documents and project proposals

When you are setting up a special programme with a range of activities over a period of time and a series of objectives, it is useful to write them into a *plan document*.

You may need a written plan to seek approval from your employers and to justify why you

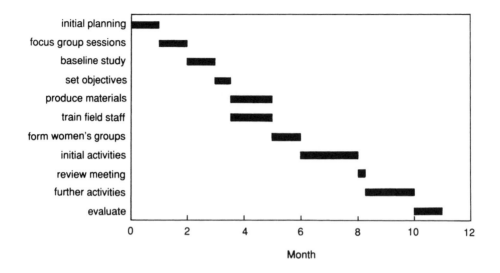

Women's Nutrition Project
Schedule of activities

Sample workplan for a 'Women's Nutrition Project'

Activities	Responsible person	Month	Indicators of achievement	Cost (US$)
1. Hold a two day workshop to orient staff on women's nutrition project.	Programme manager	Jan. 1993	Completed workshop	1 000
2. Conduct 8 focus group interviews with women in the target community.	Research officer, health education officer	Feb.	Report on focus group interviews and recommendations	3 000
3. Complete baseline study of nutrition beliefs and practices of 400 households.	Research officer, nutrition field staff	March	Completed interviews and data analysis report on baseline study	20 000
4. Produce set of measurable objectives for programme based on the data from baseline study.	Programme manager, chief nutrition officer	April	Document distributed with specific measurable objectives	300
5. Develop, pre-test and print training handbook and resource book for women on weaning foods.	Health education officer, artist	May	Copies of training handbook and leaflet printed and ready for distribution	40 000

Fig. 11.8   Workplan and bar chart: Women's Nutrition Project, schedule of activities.

should spend time on that activity and need money for equipment, transport and living expenses. However, a written plan is useful for other reasons: it makes sure that everyone is aware of what will be taking place and supports the proposed activities; it saves much time explaining to others what will actually take place; it is also a good way of allowing others to comment and make suggestions on how your plans can be improved; getting a plan approved saves time later as you will not need to obtain clearance for each separate activity.

A *project proposal* is a document outlining proposed activities and seeking permission and/or funds to proceed. A *plan* is the document that specifies what is actually going to happen. Often the same document meets both needs: before it is approved, the document is a proposal; after approval, the document is modified to take into account any suggested changes and called 'the plan'.

If you are preparing a proposal to go to a funding agency for approval it is a good idea to find out from that agency whether they have any special procedures. Often a sponsor has special requirements for information to be included in a request for funding. Sometimes they provide special forms to write the proposals. Sponsors can have different interests and these can change over time. For example, some may insist that you emphasise community participation or gender, others may be mainly interested in children.

It is helpful to meet people who have been successful in obtaining funds and ask them how they have done it. You can try to obtain copies of recent proposals that have been approved. Another useful approach is to have an informal meeting with someone from the funding agency to find out if your proposed activities fit in with their interests. You could write a short summary of what you intend to do and ask them if they think it worth your going to the trouble of preparing a detailed proposal.

If the activity you are undertaking is short and will be completed in a few days, your project proposal need only be a few pages. If your activities cover a longer period, involve large expenses and cooperation of many bodies, your

document will be longer. Guidelines for preparing a project proposal are given below. Even if you do not have to produce a written plan, it is a good idea to apply these steps. They will help you to use your time in a way that is both effective and efficient.

Preparing a project proposal

1 *Title for the programme*. The title of the project should describe the purpose of the project.
2 *Summary of plan.* Many people will not have time to read your whole plan so it is important to have a one-page summary at the beginning that lists details of proposed activities, objectives, management and budget. This should contain section or page references to the parts of the plan they deal with.
3 *Table of contents*. This should help the readers find any section of the document that they want.
4 *Statement of need or of the problem to be tackled*. You need to provide evidence in the form of reports, survey data and supporting testimonials that:
   - The problem exists in the community. You will need to include data on size of the problem – who is affected, how many are affected and whether it is increasing over time (the trend).
   - The problem is serious and having a negative effect on peoples health – causing sickness, disability or death.
   - The causes of the problem are understood. This will involve providing an analysis of the causes of the problem based on research and experience. Information presented can include the state of health services, specific policies and laws, current practices and influences on behaviours drawing on behavioural models (see Chapter 2).
   - The problem can be tackled. It is a good idea to provide examples of evaluated interventions carried out in similar communities that show that a well-planned health promotion can succeed.

- The community and other key groups perceive the problem to be serious and will support your action and become involved.
- You have the capacity, skills and experience to set up a successful programme.

5 *Mechanisms for obtaining participation of stakeholders*. This section should describe how you propose to involve all the key groups in the various stages of your programme, including defining problems, setting objectives, planning, implementation and evaluation. These include the beneficiaries in the community, relevant local groups and fieldworkers in health and other services. You should include a 'stakeholder analysis' – information on what the different stakeholders think of the problem, their views on possible solutions, their feelings about the project you are suggesting and whether they would support and become involved in your proposed programme.

6 *Specification of your objectives*. In this section you should list your objectives/targets and give reasons why each one has been selected. The objectives should be appropriate to the problem you have defined and should be achievable within the timescale you have specified.

7 *Identification of strategies*. You should explain your strategy and provide reasons for choice of methods and activities. This will involve describing:
- Health education component – who are the target group, what factors, e.g. beliefs, self-efficacy, knowledge, are you seeking to change and what methods will you use?
- Service improvements – what are the improvements in service you plan to introduce, how you will set about achieving them?
- Advocacy – what policies will you seek to influence and how will you set about doing this?

8 *Management of the activities*. Your plan should explain how you will manage your proposed activities. It is important to say who will be responsible for each activity and describe the nature of any steering group or management committee. A good way of showing this is to include an organisation diagram or 'organogram' that shows the different individuals and groups involved and the lines of responsibility and communication. It is also helpful to describe the role key persons can play in the programme and provide job specifications. As described in Chapter 4, these job specifications can also be used to explain training needs.

9 *Resources and budget*. This part of the plan should consider the needs for money, personnel, facilities, equipment and supplies. You will need to make a budget to cover the costs of the proposed tasks. The budget should cover both capital and recurrent expenditures. Capital expenditures include the cost of buying equipment, furniture and construction of buildings. Recurrent expenditures include cost of training workshops, travel and subsistence, supplies of goods such as stationery and materials, salaries of personnel, and maintenance of equipment, buildings and vehicles. You should allow for increases in prices of goods and have a contingency of at least 10% to cover unforeseen costs. There should be a description of how the funds will be managed including bookkeeping, issuing of petty cash and payment of bills.

10 *Timetable/workplan*. This part of the plan sets out the timescale for achieving the planned activities such as training, materials production and surveys. The best ways to show the sequence of activities is a bar chart (see Figure 11.8).

11 *Monitoring and evaluation*. This section describes how you will monitor and evaluate the effectiveness and efficiency of the programme. You should explain how you will obtain reliable and valid data to measure: achievement of objectives; completion of the different planned activities; use of resources and spending of budgeted funds; unforeseen benefits and disadvantages; community as well as other interested groups' views on the value of the programme. You should provide a list of the indicators of effectiveness that you will be using.

12 *Risk analysis.* In this section you identify the important assumptions you have made when planning your programme. You should also try to estimate the risk of events happening that could affect the success of your planned activities. A donor will want to check whether the assumptions you have made are justified and if you have designed your programme to take into account possible future risks.

Summary

In this chapter I have given some practical guidelines on how you can plan, manage and evaluate your communication programmes.

1 You should decide your objectives and how you will evaluate the programme at the beginning.
2 It is helpful to set out your procedures for management, community participation, monitoring and evaluation in a written plan.
3 Good communication is essential to management.
4 You should share your successes and failures with others so that the lessons learned will lead to better programmes. Why not send descriptions of your activities to the newsletters and journals listed in the Appendix?

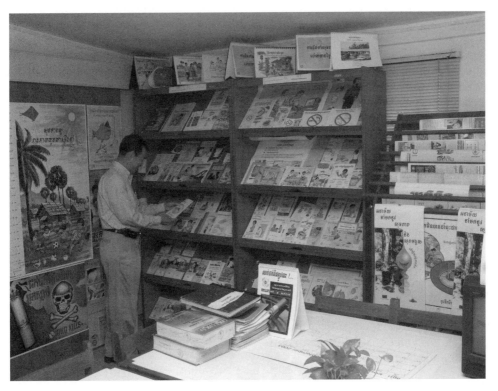

The National Centre for Health Promotion in Cambodia

Postscript

Keeping up to date in a fast-changing world

The pace of change is very fast in health promotion. We need to continually review our practices to ensure that our health promotion is effective.

- Our understanding of the influences on health and disease is improving as results of new research become available. Some practices that we may have promoted in the past may no longer be relevant, new solutions, e.g. insecticide-impregnated mosquito nets are being discovered.
- New approaches to health promotion emerge that explore different approaches to tackle difficult issues, e.g. peer education, participatory rural appraisal.
- New opportunities are being created through technology, for example the invention of the wind-up radio that does not require batteries, increased availability of video and television, the growth of low-cost regional broadcasting, video projection, the DVD format for videos, satellite transmission, e-mail and the Internet.

One of the most important movements in recent years has been that of promoting *evidence-based practice*. The movement for evidence-based practice comes from a realisation that much of what is carried out to improve health is based on tradition and fashion. We need to base our methods on what has been evaluated and shown to work. This is especially important in a new subject such as

health promotion (and its elements health communication, health education and advocacy) which is fighting for recognition as a serious discipline that deserves respect and support (and funding!).

While most people agree about the need to base practice on what has been proved to work, there are some fundamental questions that form the subject of ongoing debate, such as: What constitutes evidence? Can methods such as qualitative research provide evidence? How do you evaluate participatory and empowerment approaches? The challenge that faces us is to:

- Remember what has been done in the past but re-evaluate and assess its relevance to the situation we face today in our communities.
- Take note of new findings and be prepared to try them out if the methods seem relevant to your community. However, avoid the temptation to adopt a new approach just because it is fashionable.
- Have the courage to try out something completely new and untested if it seems appropriate to the problem you are trying to solve.
- Evaluate your work and share the results with others.

Printed sources of information

These include books, journals and newsletters.

- *Books* can include practical manuals and reviews of health topics and research findings. Books are particularly useful for manuals on how to do things. It can take two to three years to produce a book.

- *Journals* come out on a regular basis, e.g. monthly, quarterly. They usually contain papers reporting on research. The time period between writing of a paper and its appearance in print is shorter than for a book and is about 12 months. The paper has usually been subjected to a peer-review approach in which it is checked by other researchers for quality of data collection and analysis. Once it is published people can read, comment and criticise its content in follow-up papers.
- *Newsletters* are shorter publications that are often made available free to fieldworkers in developing countries. Their aim is to get information to the field as quickly as possible and the time lag between writing and publication can be as little as one month. While newsletters report on research they are not peer reviewed and do not usually give the data upon which the findings are based.

In addition a vast amount of material is produced by organisations including government ministries, international agencies, NGOs, and conference organisers. Some of these are mainly produced for their own use, others are made available for free or at a cost to others. This 'grey literature' can pose problems. It can be difficult to find out about the existence of a publication and even then it is often difficult to get hold of it. The information presented has not been subjected to any peer-review process and does not always contain enough information to evaluate the reliability and validity of the findings. It is unfortunate that many potentially valuable publications fall into this category of grey literature. Some of these eventually get published and become widely available, others become forgotten and the lessons learned never find their way into improved practice.

A list of printed resources on health promotion is given in the Appendix. I have concentrated on free newsletters and books that can easily be obtained by mail order from Teaching aids At Low Cost and Intermediate Technology Books.

The Leeds Health Education Database

This ongoing project was set up in 1997 to review the literature on health education and health communication in developing countries and prepare a database of reports of interventions that provide some evidence of impact. More than 600 documents have been reviewed but many have had to be left out of the database because the reports did not provide adequate evidence for impact. The resulting database is a collection of more than 350 reports of health promotion interventions covering a wide range of health topics and methods. The lessons learned from these evaluated programmes have been incorporated into this book. The boxes of short case studies are based on entries in the database. A detailed listing and summary of the papers in this database can be found on the web site that has been set up for this book at http://www.communicatinghealth.com

The Internet

The Internet is a network of computers all over the world. An organisation can set up a web site on a computer, and this can be accessed from anywhere in the world – provided you have a computer that can be connected to the Internet. You can look at a wide range of materials such as manuals, research reports, journals and newsletters and 'download' them to your computer to print them out and adapt for your own use.

The development of the Internet has opened up a vast resource of information. When the first edition of *Communicating Health* was released the Internet was in its infancy. A common complaint was that information was hard to obtain. The situation is very different today with millions of web sites run by every conceivable kind of organisation and individual. The problem now faced by those with Internet access is not too little information but too much!

While a valuable resource, some problems have also arisen with the Internet. There is no regulation on who can set up a site or controls on the accuracy of the information available. If you do a simple search for information on a topic, e.g. treatment for HIV/AIDS you can easily find thousands of web sites providing information on that topic with no controls on the quality or accuracy of the information. Before accepting a document from the Internet as true you need to ask the following questions:

- How responsible is the organisation that has set up the web site? Among the responsible sites are those set up by United Nations organisations (such as WHO, FAO, UNESCO, UNICEF, UNAIDS, UNFPA), the World Bank, Centers for Disease Control (Atlanta, USA) and those of NGOs with a proven track record of integrity such as Family Health International, John Hopkins University and the Communication Initiative.
- Is the information up to date? Does it take a balanced view of the subject? Does it appear to be promoting a particular point of view? Is the organisation honest about the motives for publishing the information or is there a hidden agenda? Are there commercial interests that might introduce a bias into the information provided? (For example baby milk manufacturers have been accused by IBFAN of including misleading information on their web sites.)
- Are any claims made in documents backed up by references to independent research that has been published in peer-reviewed journals?

It is always good to get different points of view. However, it is important to adopt a critical approach to *any* information you read – even from well known institutions or peer-reviewed journals.

There are many international projects that are seeking to bridge the 'digital divide' and bring the benefits of the Internet to poorer communities in the developing world. Even if you do not have access to the Internet it is still possible to get valuable information through e-mail. With e-mail you can communicate at low cost to people throughout the world. It is possible to receive electronic newsletters and join discussion groups that put you in touch with thousands of people throughout the world who can share information and help each other.

In response to the difficulties faced by fieldworkers in developing countries in gaining access to the Internet, some organisations such as TALC have started to provide extensive information on CDROMS that can be read on an ordinary computer with a CD drive.

Details of some useful web sites are provided in the Appendix. As addresses of web sites can change at short notice, you can consult the links section of the web site for this book at http://www.communicatinghealth.com for a regularly updated list of useful Internet site addresses.

Become a resource to others in your community

This can involve activities at different levels.

- providing information and resources to communities where you work;
- exchanging information and providing support to other field workers in government agencies and NGOs working in the area;
- exchanging information with organisations working at a national and international level.

One approach is to build up a small resource collection of newsletters as well as any books or teaching materials you have. You should also include in the proposal for any project you may set up, a budget to cover purchase of materials and meetings where you share your experiences with others. This is an expenditure that most sponsors will support. If you do build up a resource collection, you should distribute a catalogue to let others know what you have. You can develop a simple system for lending them out and making sure that they are returned.

Another good way of keeping in touch with others is through a regular newsletter. This can be produced simply with information on health topics and current activities. Field staff and the community can contribute through letters and articles and you can answer any questions. You can also include extracts from international newsletters on health topics.

You can keep a supply of educational materials such as leaflets, posters and visual aids in your resource centre for distribution to others. You should take care to store them in a dry and clean place so they do not get damaged. You will have to set up a system for distributing posters and educational materials to the various groups in your project.

Appendix

Suggested reading list

Books

Books available from Teaching aids At Low Cost and/or Intermediate Technology Books (see Useful Addresses on page 224)

The AIDS Handbook (3rd edition). J. Hubley 2002. Macmillan, Oxford.

Children for Health: Child-to-Child. H. Hawes and C. Scotchmer 1993. Child-to-Child Trust/UNICEF, London.

Child-to-Child, A Resource Book Part 2: Child-to-Child Activity Sheets: H. Hawes, D. Bailey and G. Bonati 1994. Child-to-Child Trust, London.

Community Based Health Care. J. Rohde and J. Wyon 2002. Management Sciences for Health, Boston.

Health into Maths. W. Gibbs and P. Mutunga 1991. Longmans, Harlow, Essex.

Health on Air. G. Adam and N. Harford 1998. Media on Air/UNAIDS, Geneva.

The Healthy Eye Activity Book – A Health Teaching Book for Primary Schools. (2nd edition) V. Francis and B. Wiafe 2001. International Centre for Eye Health, London.

Helping Health Workers Learn. D. Werner and B. Bower 1982. Hesperian Foundation, Palo Alto, California.

How to Make and Use Visual Aids. N. Harford and N. Baird 1997. Heinemann, Oxford.

Hygiene Promotion – Practical Manual for Relief and Development. S. Ferron, J. Morgan and M. O'Reilly 2000. Intermediate Technology Books, London.

Life Skills – An Active Learning Handbook for Working with Street Children. C. Hanbury 2002. Macmillan, Oxford.

Living Health Readers. Series of readers for primary schools with health themes and accompanying fact files. Macmillan, Oxford.

Participatory Learning & Action – A Trainer's Guide. J. Pretty, I. Gujit, J. Thompson and I. Scoones 1995. International Institute for Environment and Development, London.

Participatory Workshops. R. Chambers 2002. Earthscan Publications, London.

Partners in Evaluation. M.T. Feuerstein 1986. Macmillan, Oxford.

Partners in Planning. S. Rifkin and P. Pridmore 2001. Macmillan, Oxford.

Primary Health Education: B. Young and S. Durston 1997. Longmans, Harlow.

Public Health – An Action Guide to Improving Health in Developing Countries. J. Walley, J. Wright and J. Hubley 2001. Oxford University Press, Oxford.

Teaching and Learning with Visual Aids 1987. INTRAH Chapel Hill, North Carolina.

Teaching Health Care Workers. F. Abbatt and R. McMahon 1993. Macmillan, Oxford.

Training for Transformation. A. Hope and S. Timmel. Vol. 1–3 1995, Vol. 4 1999. Intermediate Technology Publications, London.

Newsletters and journals of relevance to health promotion

Newsletters marked ** are supplied free to persons from developing countries; others are available on subscription and you should write for a sample copy and their current rates.

*Baby Milk Action Newsletter.*** Baby Milk Action, 23 St Andrew's Street, Cambridge, CB2 3AX, UK

*Child-to-Child Newsletter.*** The Child-To-Child Trust, Institute of Education, University of London, 20 Bedford Way, London WC1H 0AL, UK

*Community Eye Health.*** International Eye Health Group, London School of Hygiene and Tropical Medicine, Keppel Street, London WC1E 7HT, UK

*Essential Drugs Monitor.*** WHO Action Programme on Essential Drugs and Vaccines, World Health Organization, 1211 Geneva 27, Switzerland

Health Education Research. Oxford University Press, Great Clarendon Street, Oxford OX2 6DP, UK

Health Promotion International. Oxford University Press, Great Clarendon Street, Oxford OX2 6DP, UK

International Family Planning Perspectives.** Alan Guttmacher Institute, 111 Fifth Avenue, New York, NY 10003, USA

International Quarterly of Community Health Education. Baywood Publishing Company Inc., 120 Marine St., PO Box D, Farmingdale, New York 11735, USA

Journal of Health Communication. Taylor and Francis Ltd, 11 New Fetter Lane, London EC4P 4EE, UK

Network.** Family Health International, PO Box 13950, Research Triangle Park, NC 27709, USA

Pacific AIDS Alert.** Health Programme, South Pacific Commission, BP D5,98848 Noumea, Cedex, New-Caledonia

Population Reports.** Population Information Programme, Johns Hopkins Bloomberg School of Public Health, 111 Market Place, Suite 310, Baltimore, Maryland 21201, USA

Promotion and Education (magazine of the International Union of Health Promotion Education). 2, rue Auguste Comte, 92170 Vanves, France

Sexual Health Exchange.** KIT, PO Box 95001, 1090 HA Amsterdam The Netherlands

Waterlines. ITDG Publishing Journals, c/o Portland Press, Commerce Way, Whitehall Industrial Estate, Colchester, Essex, CO2 8HP UK

Useful addresses

(See also the addresses of the agencies publishing the newsletters/journals described in the previous section.)

Academy for Educational Development, 1255 23rd Street, NW, Washington, DC, 20037, USA.

African Medical and Research Foundation (AMREF), Wilson Airport, PO Box 30125, Nairobi, Kenya

Center for Communication Programs, Johns Hopkins Bloomberg School of Public Health, 111 Market Place, Suite 310, Baltimore, Maryland 21201, USA

Centre de Formation pour la Promotion de la Santé, BP 1800, Kangu, Mayumbe, Zaire

Child-to-Child Programme, Institute of Education, University of London, 20 Bedford Way, London, WC1H 0AL, UK

Consumers International, 24, Highbury Cresent, London N5 1RX, UK

Health Action International-Europe, J. Van Lennepkade 334-T, 1053 NJ Amsterdam, The Netherlands

Health Education Unit, Leeds Metropolitan University, Leeds LS1 3HE, UK

Healthlink Worldwide, Cityside, 40 Adler Street, London E1 1EE, UK

Intermediate Technology Books, 103–105 Southampton Row, London, WC1B 4HL, UK

International Baby Foods Action Network, IBFAN, c/o GIFA, CP 157, 1211 Geneva 19, Switzerland

International Reference Centre for Community Water Supply and Sanitation Programmes, PO Box 93190, 2509 AD The Hague, Netherlands

Teaching aids At Low Cost (TALC), PO Box 49, St Albans, Herts AL1 5TX, UK

UNESCO. Unit for Cooperation with UNICEF and WFP, UNESCO, 7 Place de Fontenoy, 75700 Paris, France

UNICEF, 866 UN Plaza, United Nations, New York NY 10017, USA

World Health Organization, 1211 Geneva 27, Switzerland

Internet web sites

Addresses for web sites can change without notice. Below are listed some important web sites that are unlikely to change. A comprehensive list of web sites is provided on the web site for this book (see below).

Agencies

UNAIDS (http://www.unaids.com)
UNICEF (http://www.unicef.org/)
UNESCO (http://www.unesco.org)
WHO International Headquarters (http://www.who.ch)
PAHO – WHO regional office for the Americas (http://www.paho.org)
Centers for Disease Control, Atlanta, USA (http://www.cdc.gov)

Networks

International Union of Health Promotion and Education (http://www.iuhpe.org)
One World Network (http://www.oneworld.net)

Resources

Communications Initiative (http://www.comminit.com)
Johns Hopkins Communication Project (http://www.jhuccp.org)
American Public Health Association (http://www.apha.org)

The web site for this book

A web site has been set up especially to support this book at the following address:

http://www.communicatinghealth.com

The web site will contain:
• full details of all the case studies presented in the book;
• updates on any key developments;
• resources that can be used by trainers to accompanying the book including PowerPoint presentations and participatory learning exercises;
• an extensive set of links to relevant web sites on the Internet that will be regularly updated.

Index